...und Medea war eine Ärztin

Berliner Beiträge zur Literatur- und Kulturgeschichte

Herausgegeben von
Irmela von der Lühe und Gail K. Hart

Band 1

PETER LANG
Frankfurt am Main · Berlin · Bern · Bruxelles · New York · Oxford · Wien

Magdalena Tarnawska

...und Medea war eine Ärztin

Constructions of Femininity in Public Debates about Medical Education for Women in Germany and Austria between 1870 and 1910

PETER LANG
Internationaler Verlag der Wissenschaften

Bibliographic Information published by the Deutsche Nationalbibliothek
The Deutsche Nationalbibliothek lists this publication in the Deutsche Nationalbibliografie; detailed bibliographic data is available in the internet at <http://www.d-nb.de>.

ISSN1862-815X
ISBN 978-3-631-56396-0

www.peterlang.de

Acknowledgments

First and foremost, I would like to express my immense gratitude to Professor Gail Hart, without whom this publication would not have been possible. It was Professor Hart who encouraged me to revise my dissertation written in the Department of German at the University of California, Irvine, and submit it for publication. She proofread and provided crucial feedback on multiple drafts of the manuscript and suggested the title for this book. Professor Hart has been an exceptional mentor and dedicated supporter of my research and was extremely helpful in crystallizing many of my arguments and deepening my critical analysis of archival material. The intellectual support and enthusiasm she continuously expressed about my work were among the highlights of my writing process. My deepest appreciation goes to Professor Jens Rieckmann, who patiently and generously guided and supported me during the crucial time of my dissertation research and writing, and to Professor Meredith Lee, whose insightful comments led me to sharpen the analytical lens of my arguments. I wish to extend an expression of appreciation to Prof. Dr. Irmela von der Lühe for helpful advice during the writing and editing process. Special thanks go to Dr. Christa Franke and Professor Jennifer Terry for inspiring conversations. The major work for this book has been completed during my graduate studies at the University of California, Irvine, and I want to thank all my professors, mentors, and colleagues for their intellectual and emotional support. I am especially indebted to Professor Glenn Levine for continuous encouragement and assistance. I am very grateful to Judith Magyar for proofreading the manuscript and being always available for additional help and advice. My thanks go to my friends who helped countless times in many different ways: Inge Aures, Jeanne Batalova, Céline Jacquemin, and Gosia Wąsik. Generous financial support was provided by the University of California, Irvine, for the archival research in Germany, without which this book would not have been possible: I was awarded a Summer Dissertation Fellowship by the Department of German in 2000 and a Summer Dissertation Fellowship by the School of Humanities in 2001. In 2003 I also received a German Academic Exchange Service (DAAD) Scholarship, which enabled me to complete the final stages of my archival research. The University of California Regents' Dissertation Fellowship in 2003 allowed me to finish the writing of my dissertation. I want to thank DePauw University in Greencastle, Indiana, for a generous publishing subvention. Above all I want to express my immense gratitude to my family for their unconditional love, caring, and support: my loving husband, who always believed in my success; my father and Hella, who always cared and were available to help; my mother, my grandmother, and Rysiu, who were always supportive and proud of me; and my wonderful brother, who could make me laugh during tough times. I also dedicate this book in memory of my grandmother Bunia, who loved me so much; my grandfather Władzio, who introduced me to the world of art; and my grandfather Marian, who told me countless stories. I would not be who I am today without you. Thank you for everything.

Table of Contents

Introduction 9

CHAPTER 1 The Struggle for Women's Admission to Medical Schools: Politics of the Female Body 23
1.1 Introduction: Historical Overview 23
1.2 Position on Female Education Peculiar to Germany and Austria 32
1.3 Major Arguments in the Debate about Women's Admission to Medical Schools 38
1.3.1 Morality 39
1.3.2 Reproduction 43
1.3.3 Economics 44
1.3.4 Science and Nature 46
1.3.5 Tradition and Social Control 49
1.4 Female Responses to Kirchhoff's Survey 51

CHAPTER 2 Alleged Consequences of the Brain Structure and of the Anatomy of the Female Body 57
2.1 Introduction: Texts and Arguments Opening the Debates in Germany 57
2.2 The Female Brain 58
2.3 The Correlation between (Pseudo) Scientific Pamphlets and Political Decisions 63
2.4 Other Anatomical Differences 65
2.5 Gender-Specific Division of Labor 68
2.6 Class and Gender 72
2.7 Dichotomy of Reason and Emotion and Other Gender-Specific Qualities 78

CHAPTER 3 The Female Body and Regulatory Practices in the Public and Private Space 83
3.1 Introduction: Intersections of Space, Gender, and Class 83
3.2 One Female Sex and Multiple Gender Types 86
3.3 Eduard Albert and the Lack of Scientific Objectivity 99
3.4 The Female Body as an Object of Aesthetic and Sensual Pleasure 103
3.5 The Female Body in the Private Realm 111
3.6 The Public Space of the University 117

CHAPTER 4 The Woman's Reproductive Body and Scientific Production of Knowledge 121
4.1 Introduction: Conflicting Views on Female Reproductive Physiology 121
4.2 Max Runge's *Das Weib in seiner geschlechtlichen Eigenart* 123
4.3 The Question of Knowledge Production 127
4.4 Different Modes of Knowledge 130
4.5 The Reproductive Body 134
4.6 Modes of Control of the Female Body 139

CHAPTER 5 Against Pornographic Imagination: the Autonomous Female Body 143
5.1 Introduction: Reactions to Paul Julius Möbius 143
5.2 Möbius' Text as a Cultural Manifesto 148
5.3 Pornographic Imagination 152
5.4 Möbius' Text as an Expression of Pornographic Imagination ... 156
5.5 From Nature to Culture: Progress of Civilization 162
5.6 Feminist Interpretation of Biological Data 171
5.7 From *Weib* to *Frau*: the New Woman 174

Conclusion 179
Works Cited 181

Introduction

Medicine [...] often categorizes problems fundamentally social in origin as biological or personal deficits, and in so doing smothers the impulse for social change which could offer the only serious resolution.

Evan Stark and Anne Flitcraft[1]

At any given time, the more powerful side will create an ideology suitable to help maintain its position and to make this position acceptable to the weaker one. In this ideology the differentness of the weaker one will be interpreted as inferiority, and it will be proven that these differences are unchangeable, basic or God's will. It is the function of such an ideology to deny or conceal the existence of struggle.

Karen Horney[2]

In an article "Down with Love," published in the popular magazine *Elle* in May 2004, Steve Friedman tells his readers a number of anecdotes that are supposed to illustrate a new trend in US society—a lack of interest on the part of women in forming committed relationships with men. The article concludes as follows: "So a lot of men want to cook, to cuddle, to have company on the futon. Does this make us [men] the 'new women'? Maybe. I can live with that. [...] What about the women who [...] view the opposite sex as amusing toys, conniving enemies, or duplicitous tricksters, then act accordingly? Such women, I would submit, are the new men" (Friedman 168). Additionally, the author feels compelled to include a statement about the connection between gender roles and biological determination ("Biology may no longer be destiny" [Friedman 166]) and to give his article more validity by quoting "the director of the Evolutionary Psychology Lab at Florida Atlantic University" (Friedman 168). Although the article does not provide any kind of sophisticated analysis of new trends in contemporary heterosexual relationships, it clearly illustrates certain anxieties in relation to unconventional gender models. It also demonstrates a compulsive need to label behaviors and qualities as gender-specific, feminine or masculine. Even though in this article the conventional gender roles are turned upside down, they are still as rigid as the traditional ones. Furthermore, while the allegedly new male characteristics are displayed in a positive light, a negative twist is given to the qualities attributed to women. The fear of women turning into "men" thematized by the article is not new. It had been raised and fiercely discussed more than a hundred years ago, in a

1 Qtd. in Kohler Riessman 49.
2 Qtd. in Ussher 255.

tone quite similar to the one used by Friedman. While discussing nineteenth-century medical texts, a contemporary historian Katrin Schmersahl, for example, pointed to an argument very similar to the one implied by Friedman, that is, that "[p]ositiv konnotierte 'männliche' Eigenschaften verkehren sich bei Frauen in ihr Gegenteil und führen zur – oftmals sexuell konnotierten – Herrschaft der Frau und zur Versklavung des Mannes" (328-29). I address the link between contemporary fears of crossing gender boundaries and anxieties manifested a century ago because this connection demonstrates the continuing and contested nature of processes involved in construction and representation of gender identities. Looking back at shifts in the understanding of femininity and masculinity over the course of history allows us better to understand the mechanisms of these constructions operating today.

This book explores a shift in gender politics in Germany and Austria between 1870 and 1910 that was initiated, as I argue, by the struggle of middle-class women to gain access to higher education. Excluding women from universities was based on popular and (pseudo) scientific notions of femininity according to which women were irrational by nature and not capable of critical or analytical thinking; woman's primary functions were to serve her husband, to give birth, and to rear children; and child bearing and intellectual development were seen as mutually exclusive. Supporters of higher education for women questioned these notions of femininity that were based on certain assumptions about women's sexuality, their "nature," and their bodies. Consequently, at the core of the discussion regarding admission of women to higher education was the normative discourse on the female body and sexuality. I focus on the public debates about admission of women to medical schools because I believe that they provide a unique insight into gender politics at the end of the nineteenth century for the following reasons. First, medical discourse played a major role in defining biological differences between the sexes and in determining gender roles in society. Second, knowledge about the anatomy and functions of the human body was perceived as inappropriate for young middle-class women. Finally, the relationship between a physician and a patient involved a power relationship. Hence, the medical field was the most contested arena of struggle between different gender ideologies. The first part of this book's title refers to an extreme example of the anxiety that a female physician evoked in many opponents of medical education for women. "...und Medea war eine Ärztin" is a quotation from an article "Weibliche Ärzte" published in 1907 under the pseudonym Avicenna in the journal *Die Fackel*, in which the author explains a woman's desire for medical education as an expression of her perverted sexual drive.[3] Although this article is a very extreme example of the general societal resistance to women entering the medical profession as physicians, it gives a glimpse into more general social fears connected to women's struggle for higher education. Medea, best known for

3 This article will be discussed extensively in Chapter Three.

slaying her children as an act of vengeance against their father, is the most unmotherly of mothers in the traditional telling of the myth. In fact, she is a monster–not a woman. The annihilation of the motherly love in the Medea-myth gives this heroine a monstrous dimension. Within the patriarchal order, this monstrous dimension is deepened by Medea's lack of subordination to male authority; she deceives and abandons her father, kills her brother, and turns against the father of her children when he decides to marry another woman. Medea's attributes, projected onto female physicians, infuse these women with monstrous qualities; they become something that the society at large resists and fears. Indeed, many opponents of medical education for women perceived a female physician as an individual who did not adhere to social norms and conventions and was, for that reason, unpredictable and potentially dangerous.

To examine how the popular understanding of femininity shifted in the German-speaking society as a result of women's demands for access to the university, I analyze public discussions about education carried out in the press and (pseudo) scientific texts written by physicians and university professors, as well as reactions to these texts mainly by German and Austrian women writers and activists. My objective is to demonstrate how these intellectuals attempted to negotiate new roles for women by responding directly to opponents of female education. These reactions are important because, in addition to engaging in the negotiation of new gender roles, they document the emergence of a new female subjectivity. They also challenge the institutional, cultural, and social structures of the time. I argue that these early feminists attempted to redefine popular understandings of gender and sexuality in their struggle for equal rights, such as access to education and employment. Their active participation in the public discussion surrounding female nature gave them the opportunity to uncover, influence, and alter the politics of the female body. In addition, it had a direct impact on legislative decisions sanctioning female presence at the university. Hence, the importance of female responses cannot be underestimated. In addition, in my analysis of the debates about medical education for women, I explore the role of medicine in creating gendered subjects. I also examine the intersections of science, medicine, and popular culture and the ways in which popular concepts of gender differences influenced scientific investigation. The statement by Evan Stark and Anne Flitcraft at the beginning of this introduction accurately characterizes the situation in the late nineteenth century. Physicians and medical scientists agitating against higher education for women in Germany and Austria, indeed, branded the social origins of the struggle as pathological.[4]

In this book I use the term "femininity" to refer to a set of characteristics widely believed to constitute femaleness (Morawski). This set of characteristics is historically and culturally specific. Discussions about femininity and representations of femininity create the very meaning of the term. In the context of the public

4 Schmersahl develops a similar argument throughout her book. The core of this argument is "Pathologisierung nonkonformer sozialer Verhaltensweisen" (Schmersahl 15).

discussion about the admission of women to medical schools, three different notions of femininity emerge. I refer to these as passive body without voice (corresponding to the traditional concept of womanhood as confined to the private sphere), active voice without body (relating to the symbolic transgression of the public space by female writers), and active body with voice (being physically present at a university and demonstrating that leaving the private sphere itself is a statement about women's role in society). Conventional male theories of femininity that I discuss are based on the dichotomy between a dynamic, active, and aggressive man and a passive, submissive, and receptive woman. In this gender model, woman is denied autonomy and agency. Hence, she becomes merely a passive body without a voice. Many female intellectuals and activists agitated for gender equality by writing newspaper articles and books, by responding to the opponents of higher education for women, and by discrediting their arguments. They spoke up and forced others to acknowledge the female voice, but they did not transgress public space in a physical way. Hence, they became an active voice without a body. Female students acted upon the demand to gain access to higher education. They manifested their belief in gender equality through physical presence at the university. Hence they became an active body with a voice. This book illustrates the interplay of these three notions of femininity. In addition, I demonstrate that the opponents of higher education for women perceived femininity as essential and nature-given. If altered, it would produce abnormal and pathological qualities. Many of the supporters, in contrast, understood the notion of femininity as socially constructed and challenged these conventional and limited ways of looking at gender identity.

The quotation from Karen Horney that precedes this introduction emphasizes the ideological foundation of social inequality, a question that is relevant to my analysis. Many physicians and medical scientists opposing female education attempted to deliver such an ideological foundation.[5] They gave public lectures and published texts portraying the anatomy and/or physiology of the female body as a major obstacle on the road leading to higher education. They depicted women as being limited by their bodies, not able to overcome the limitations imposed by anatomical structures and physiological functions, the most important being menstruation and pregnancy. Men, on the other hand, were not limited by their bodies; their bodily functions did not impose any restrictions on their lives. While man's ability to think allowed him to transcend the physical boundary by participating in the spiritual and intellectual realm, a woman was trapped and bound by the functioning of her reproductive organs and limited to the physical aspects of her body. Precisely because of her physiology, she could not transcend the physical realm. Such (pseudo) scientific views mirrored the popular obsession with gender distinctions in the nineteenth century. Male and female personality traits, intellectual abilities, even types of behavior were derived from two body parts, the uterus in

5 This is also an argument that Schmersahl develops throughout her book. See, for example, Schmersahl 60; 111-112; 302.

the case of women, and the brain in the case of men.[6] Both organs became the focal points in the discussions surrounding gender issues and were believed to be main signifiers of womanhood and manhood.[7] The focus on the male brain and the female uterus can also be understood on a symbolic level as a manifestation of the dichotomy between the mental/spiritual (cognitive function) and the physical (childbearing) realm. Within this framework, the focus of arguments against women's medical education changed over the years. While brain research seemed to occupy opponents of women's higher education in the 1870s, the 1890s had a greater interest in female sexuality. Nevertheless, a correlation between the two had always constituted the core of the arguments against higher education for women.[8]

This book is, by the nature of the research questions I had asked, interdisciplinary. The secondary literature I consulted and the scholarship I included in my arguments span multiple disciplines: German social history, history of medicine and education, women's and gender studies, German literature and cultural studies. Although the history of women's admission to higher education and the history of the women's movement provide necessary background for my investigation, they are not the subject of this book. Nor do I investigate biographies of women students, writers, and activists. Instead, as the title of this book suggests, the main focus of my research lies in various constructions of femininity rooted in competing gender ideologies. My primary goal is to document a changing social awareness relating to gender roles and the emergence of a new self-understanding in the texts by several middle-class women. Investigating contested social terrains gives us insight into various practices and ideologies determining social reality and, above all, into the mechanisms of change. The debates concerned with higher education for women carried out in various publications and lectures at the end of the nineteenth century proved to be sensitive indicators of changes in social consciousness[9] regarding gender roles. The texts published at the time recorded

6 Referring to Anna Bergmann, Schmersahl writes: "ein Orgen – das Gehirn – [wurde] zum Repräsentanten eines gesellschaftlichen Prinzips, nämlich der Rationalität, die a priori als 'männlich' galt" (79). Schmersahl also argues that "[d]ie Fixierung auf das Gehirn war [...] von Vorteil, weil mit ihr – im Gegensatz etwa zur Gynäkologie, die den weiblichen Geschlechtscharakter aus den weiblichen Generationsorganen und -funktionen ableitet und von hier aus das Sozialverhalten von Frauen kontrollierte – auch das soziale Verhalten von Männern medizinisch erfaßbar wurde" (64).

7 The scientific fixation on the brain and the uterus might be explained by a relatively new trend in nineteenth-century medicine. As Schmersahl pointed out "[i]m 19. Jahrhundert setzten sich zunehmend ein an den einzelnen Organen orientiertes Denken und eine spezialistisch-technische Expertenkultur durch" (195).

8 The connection between brain research and research of female sexuality receives an interesting dimension in Schmersahl's book. She points to professional competition between psychiatrists and neurologists on the one hand and gynecologists on the other (Schmersahl 191; 206-211).

9 Romana Weiershausen argues that the struggle for higher education for women created "für die Literatur [...] neue[n] Imaginationsraum" (12) that became "Schau[platz] institutioneller

traces of competing ideologies as well as social anxieties and emerging new possibilities.

The recent scholarship that intersects most directly with my research includes the following publications: Helga Mae Thorson's dissertation, "Re-Negotiating Borders: Responses of German and Austrian Middle-Class Women Writers to Medical Discourse on Sex, Gender, and Sexuality at the Turn of the Century" (1996); Katrin Schmersahl's *Medizin und Geschlecht. Zur Konstruktion der Kategorie Geschlecht im medizinischen Diskurs des 19. Jahrhunderts* (1998); Patricia M. Mazón's *Gender and the Modern Research University. The Admission of Women to German Higher Education, 1865-1914* (2003); and Romana Weiershausen's *Wissenschaft und Weiblichkeit. Die Studentin in der Literatur der Jahrhundertwende* (2004). A brief discussion of these publications will allow me to situate my book within the most recent scholarship and demonstrate how it complements that research on the one hand and how it problematizes certain issues on the other.

Thorson discusses the notion of borderlands in relation to gender and race and analyzes the concept of the "third sex" (hermaphrodite) and of the "mixed-race" body. She also examines the discussion of hysteria and analyzes the role that the notion of female and male hysterics played in the construction of gender and normative sexuality. While Thorson primarily discusses women's reactions to broader questions pertaining to gender and race and includes literary works in her analysis, I focus on women's responses to specific texts written by physicians relating to the question of medical education for women.

Schmersahl examines intersections of medicine, gender politics, and the social order. Specifically, she looks at the degree to which medical texts and theories were rooted in the ideology of difference in regard to the sexes and in what way they were constitutive of the existing gender order in society.[10] Her investigation is based on the Foucaultian premise that medicine in particular and natural sciences in general constitute a time-specific and changeable system of knowledge[11] that is embedded in a complex nexus of power (Schmersahl 11). Hence, medicine does not just record and describe the "facts" it discovers, but rather produces a regulatory system that justifies and co-creates a particular social order (Schmersahl 11). Drawing on scholarship by Claudia Honegger, Barbara Duden, and Thomas Laqueur, specifically on their theories about the role that medicine played in "Ausformulierung, Legitimierung und Durchsetzung der Geschlechtscharaktere und deren Bedeutung für medizinische Theoriebildung" (12),

---

und ideologischer Kämpfe" (Greenblatt qtd. in Weiershausen 12). Literature, Weiershausen continues, has a double role; it is both "indicator" of and "factor" in social changes (12).

10 "Es muß zum einen danach gefragt werden, inwiefern medizinische Theorien durch das Postulat der Geschlechterdifferenz strukturiert wurden. Zum anderen muß herausgestellt werden, welchen Anteil die Medizin an der Herstellung der Geschlechterordnung hatte" (Schmersahl, Vorwort).

11 "ein historisch bedingtes und variables Wissenssystem" (Schmersahl, Vorwort).

Schmersahl investigates "die geschlechtsspezifischen Dimensionen medizinischer Theorien" (12) and how they contributed to "Ausdifferenzierung der Ärzteschaft, ihrer gesellschaftlichen Reputation und zur Konstruktion und Etablierung bürgerlicher Normen" in German-speaking countries between 1800 and 1912 (12). In her analysis of the nineteenth-century medical discourse, Schmersahl stresses its overt misogyny and points to a reciprocal relationship between medical theories and gender-specific norms of social conduct. She emphasizes, for example, that behaviors not conforming to the established social norms were often medicalized and categorized in terms of disorders (104).[12] Schmersahl ends her book by sketching the realm that has opened up for academic investigation: reactions to the medical discourse of the nineteenth century. She points to additional research questions logically following her work and still to be answered by future scholarship.[13] This book takes up the questions concerned with the impact of medical theories on women's lives as well as the questions pertaining to the existence, origins, authorship, and influence of the counter-discourse. On the one hand, I continue Schmersahl's investigation of the misogynist attitudes inherent in the (pseudo) scientific writings. On the other hand, however, I explore the counter-discourse generated by the medical texts.

Mazón focuses on the issue of higher education for women in Germany between 1865 and 1914 and analyzes the structure of the German research university and its ideological foundations. The notion of "academic citizenship" (Mazón 3) proves crucial for her investigation as she attempts to provide an answer to the question "[w]hy were women considered antithetical to the very essence of the university?" (3). Analyzing the structure of the nineteenth-century German university, Mazón is concerned with the role that "university standards, roles, and expectations" played in the debates about potential female students and with "an understanding of how gender helped to construct academic roles and institutional authority in Imperial Germany" (12). While analyzing the notion of "academic citizenship" that was male by its very definition (19-49) and discussing the attempts made by women's organizations and individual activists to grant women access to higher education and employment in the context of the nineteenth-century "woman question" (50-84), Mazón sees the debate about higher education for women as a "clash between the rhetoric of the woman question and that of academic citizenship" (17; 85-114). Finally she gives an overview of the legislation concerning women's admission to the German universities (115-151),

12 See also the statement by Evan Stark and Anne Flitcraft at the beginning of the introduction.

13 Schmersahl suggests the following questions: "Inwiefern rekurrierten andere zeitgenössische Diskurse auf den medizinischen? Wie wirkte dieser sich konkret im Leben einzelner Menschen aus? Gab es Gegendiskurse? Und wenn ja, von wem, wie und wo wurden diese geführt? [...] [W]elchen Einfluß [hatten] medizinische Theorien auf das Leben und die Lebensentwürfe von Frauen [...]? Kannten Frauen den medizinischen Diskurs über ihr Geschlecht und erkannten sie dessen misogynen Gehalt? Inwiefern und wie setzten sie sich damit auseinander?" (Schmersahl 347).

analyzes literary representations of female students (152-176), and examines autobiographical texts by women who had entered academic fields (176-223). Mazón explores the debate about higher education for women as "a cultural artifact" (4) that gives insight into "the larger worlds of German society and politics" (4), which is also my approach. However, while Mazón looks at the issue of higher education as such through the prism of "academic citizenship" and the question of "bourgeois masculine identity" (86), I focus on the notion and the status of the female body in the debates about admission of women to medical education. In addition, I use the debates about higher education primarily to illustrate gender politics in the late nineteenth century. Central to Mazón's argument is the claim that while the question of higher education for women was approached by the supporters of the issue as "a solution to a social problem," the opponents, especially university authorities and professors, perceived it as "a threat to the idea of academic citizenship" (Mazón 86). Discussing the educational demands of the German women's movement, Mazón emphasizes the different strategies women activists used to campaign for higher education (50-84). She argues that women tried to establish grounds for their inclusion in the "academic citizenship" not by redefining femininity, but by "constructing a new way of belonging, a new definition of membership in realms long closed to their sex" (Mazón 84). My arguments, conversely, focus on women's attempts to redefine the prevalent notion of femininity.

Mazón divides the German women's movement of the nineteenth century into two factions: one arguing for women's rights on the basis of women's equality with men, the other attempting to reach the same goal by emphasizing the differences between the sexes (53). She also refers to a common scholarly approach among contemporary historians to attribute "the triumph of an ideology of 'difference' over that of 'equality'" to the German women's movement (53). Mazón continues by noting that, in these approaches, "difference and equality mean two rhetorical strategies, usually seen as mutually exclusive, with which women could argue for the improvement of their condition" (53).[14] Later, however, she makes the issue problematic by pointing out that activists usually seen as advocates of one of the factions "shared a whole range of assumptions about gender identity and possibilities for reform" (Mazón 53). Precisely the emphasis on this range of assumptions in writings by several nineteenth-century activists will be central to my line of argument. Regardless of whether these women emphasized difference or equality of the sexes, they all participated in the molding of the notion of femininity into new shapes. In this book, I am not as much concerned with emphasizing the differences and similarities between various arguments

14 See also Mazón's footnote 10 (53; 241). Referring to Margit Twellmann, Weiershausen also emphasizes that arguments rooted in the ideology of difference between the sexes were prevalent in the German women's movement. Therefore, instead of campaigning for full equality (which few women did), many activists demanded equality only in certain areas for which women were seen as suited on the basis of their "nature" (Weiershausen 40).

within the women's movement or with labeling the activists as adhering to certain ideologies as I am with focusing on newly emerging notions of femininity. In addition, I believe that the debate about higher education for women as a whole demonstrated a phenomenon that was very new to the social consciousness of nineteenth-century society, namely that gender identity is an object of negotiation and not a nature-given entity. Not single arguments of selected individuals, but the participation of a substantial number of middle-class women in the debate contributed to this change.[15] Hence, the act of middle-class women claiming voice in the public realm was of great importance. Here, I agree with Mazón who claims that "the nineteenth-century bourgeois women's movement was about women learning to speak in public" (50). Not only through their arguments but also through the act of speaking up and reacting to medical texts and theories, these women managed to destabilize popular and scientific concepts of femininity.

Weiershausen focuses on the female student as a new literary figure that had been introduced into German literature at the end of the nineteenth century and explores the functions this figure played in various literary texts.[16] She is interested in finding out "wie sich im Fall der Studentin [...] [das] Verhältnis zwischen Darstellung eines aktuellen sozialgeschichtlichen Phänomens und seiner (Neu-) Imagination und Inszenierung im literarischen Raum ausprägte" (13). Drawing primarily on Michel Foucault's discourse theory, on its appropriation for literary theory by Jürgen Link and Ursula Link-Heer (Weiershausen 23-24), as well as on Stephen Greenblatt's understanding of literary texts as "Schauplätze institutioneller und ideologischer Kämpfe" (Weiershausen 27), Weiershausen analyzes literary texts within their sociohistorical and time-specific philosophical context and looks at literature as a special type of discourse[17] which, to a very high degree, integrates elements of other discourses (25). The struggle for the admission of women to higher education as well as various reactions of the society to the appearance of the first female students constitute for Weiershausen's arguments a necessary sociohistorical framework (Weiershausen 20). Within this framework,

---

15 While referring to the public campaign by the women's movement, Mazón mentions that "petitions were another way of keeping the subject of the *Frauenstudium* before the public" (97). She also refers to James Albisetti who "has noted, petitions were unsuccessful in parliament but stimulated public discussion nonetheless" (97).

16 Weiershausen analyzes the following literary texts: Käthe Schirmacher's *Die Liebertad* (1891), Ilse Frapan's *Wir Frauen haben kein Vaterland* (1899) and *Arbeit* (1903), Ella Mensch's *Auf Vorposten* (1903), Lou Andreas-Salomé's *Fenitschka* (1898), Erwin Guido Kolbenheyer's *Montsalvasch* (1912), Gerhart Hauptmann's *Einsame Menschen* (1891), and Elsa Bernstein's *Dämmerung* (1893). In addition, Weiershausen included a complete bibliography of literary texts published between 1881 and 1910 which feature a female student (273-275).

17 Weiershausen uses the term discourse as "Ausdruck von Machtbeziehungen [...], die [...] soziale Wirklichkeit konstituieren" and, therefore, "müssen in ihrer historischen Wandelbarkeit und in ihrer Wechselwirkung mit konkreten sozialen Bedingungen wahrgenommen werden" (Weiershaisen 24).

literary texts with female students as protagonists "entfalten ihre soziale Energie gerade vor dem Hintergrund der sozialpolitischen Kontroverse" (Weiershausen 28) and interact in various ways with the sociopolitical background from which they had emerged (Weiershausen 28).[18] The appearance of female students was without a doubt, as Weiershausen claims, "Anlaß, Weiblichkeit neu and anders zu diskutieren" (265). The female student has also been for my exploration a crucial figure through which "die bislang dominierende Entgegensetzung [...] von Wissenschaft und Weiblichkeit in grundlegender Weise in Bewegung geriet" (Weiershausen 261) and a figure that became "Testfall [...] für die Weiblichkeitsbilder, die um die Jahrhundertwende dominant [waren]" (266). Through the figure of the female student, Weiershausen writes, a question "nach dem *Wesen des Weibes*" transformed into a question "nach der Einordnung einer aus dem Rahmen fallenden Figur in bereits vorliegende Weiblichkeitsmuster" (265). This is a valid claim, especially in relation to opponents of higher education for women. However, I also contend that the question "nach dem *Wesen des Weibes*" put forward by scientists and physicians was transformed into a question of self-discovery for many women as reflected by the essays analyzed in this book. While Weiershausen looks at the female student as a literary figure and explores this figure's functions and its "subversive[s] Potential" (260) within literary texts, I am interested in tracing the development of a new self-understanding in women's non-fictional writings, specifically in their direct responses to (pseudo) scientific misogynistic texts. Although I agree with Weiershausen that literature is, of course, a more or less direct response to the sociohistorical situation and that some women used literary texts "um ihre programmatische Position narrativ zu entfalten und das wissenschaftliche Studium der Frau am Beispiel handelnder und

---

18 The texts by Schirmacher, Mensch, and Frapan are primarily "Beiträge zur sozialpolitischen Debatte über das Frauenstudium und zu einer davon ausgehenden Kritik an gesellschaftlichen Zuständen" (Weiershausen 63). In contrast, the texts by Andreas-Salomé and Kolbenheyer are understandable "erst im Kontext des philosophisch-weltanschaulichen Diskurses der Zeit" (Weiershausen 264). Regardless of the scope and depth of the intertextual dialogue in which these literary works participate, all of them, according to Weiershausen, tackle the question "nach der Weiblichkeit der Studentin" (Weiershausen 162; see also 266). Texts by Schirmacher, Mensch, and Frapan demonstrate that a pursuit of academic education by women does not diminish their femininity (Weiershausen 139). Andreas-Salomé goes even further, as Weiershausen claims. The main character of Andreas-Salomé's *Fenitschka*, the female student, "reprasentiert eine höherentwickelte Weiblichkeit" (Weiershausen 139). For Erwin Guido Kolbenheyer, the female student fails as a woman (which for him means wife and mother) and his novel is "die endgültige Diskreditierung der Studentin" (Weiershausen 173). For Bernstein, the university-educated woman ophthalmologist is "aufgeklärter Mensch, der zu einer vollkommenen Liebe fähig ist" (Weiershausen 259). In Gerhard Hauptmann's *Einsame Menschen*, the female student is depicted as "ganz weiblich" from the very beginning (Weiershausen 266). Weiershausen, argues, that in all these texts, the female student becomes "Vertreterin der modernen Zeit" (214). While this development is depicted as positive in most of the texts, for Kolbenheyer the female student is "degeneriertes Zivilisationsprodukt" (Weiershausen 259).

reflektierender Figuren lebensweltlich zu konkretisieren" (268-69), I was interested in obtaining much more literally than literarily direct answers to the research questions I had asked. Choosing essays and non-fictional writings gave me that opportunity.

In addition to designating a genre of writing, an essay is an effort or a trial, an experiment in thinking and re-thinking. Responses to (pseudo) scientific misogynistic texts in the form of essays and other non-fictional writings became for many women an attempt to test and to think through new notions of femininity and to re-define their own position in society in a very direct way. These essays deal with questions of knowledge, gender, autonomy, and power in very complex ways, and they document "die Umbruchszeit" (Weiershausen 261; Schmersahl 302), as much as the literary texts do.

This book can be situated in the field of German cultural studies and characterized as a discourse analysis within a framework of social constructivism. I examine a variety of discourses created by medicine, science, popular culture, and early feminist resistance to male-dominated public life. In addition, my work draws on a theoretical perspective that understands the historically and culturally specific construction of gender identity. Concepts that guide my thinking here include, but are not limited to, Judith Butler's notion of the unstable and performative character of gender identity, Michel Foucault's analysis of the discursive formation of body and sexuality, and Anne Fausto-Sterling's view of science as reinforcing the dominant ideology. Although my work has been influenced by a variety of theoretical approaches, I have not adopted any particular theory or set of theories in an absolute or inflexible way.

My research has been guided by the following questions: How is gender constructed in the texts/arguments opposing higher education of women? What do these texts tell us about scientific, medical, and popular constructions of femininity at the end of the nineteenth century? In what way do these (pseudo) scientific models reflect cultural/popular notions of gender differences? How do women intervene in the process of (pseudo) scientific knowledge production and dissemination? How do women writers and feminist activists destabilize the prevalent notions of femininity? How do they construct alternative gender models? How do these intellectuals negotiate new understanding of femininity? Although I do not claim that I have answered these questions completely and definitively, I believe that this book illuminates the plurality of voices involved in the construction and representation of gendered cultural experience in Germany and Austria and that it helps us better understand the notions of femininity operating in late-nineteenth-century discourses.

In the course of this book I investigate the foundation, development, and stages of the debate regarding female admission to medical schools. I discuss five major texts by physicians and opponents of women's entrance into the medical profession as well as women's responses to them. I chose these particular texts because they generated the greatest number of women's responses and were very popular at the time. These texts also denote four major stages in the struggle for women's admission to higher education and in the development of public opinion in matters of gender equality. All these stages mirror a gradual change in the social consciousness regarding the notion of femininity and reflect a process in which women negotiate different roles for themselves, gain a new self-understanding, and question the existing institutional structures of society. In my discussion of the struggle for women's admission to medical schools, I focus on all stages of this debate. Each stage is marked by a different text opposing female medical education and the responses it generated. The earliest texts, Theodor Bischoff's *Das Studium und die Ausübung der Medizin durch Frauen* (1872) and Wilhelm Waldeyer's "Das Studium der Medizin und die Frauen" (1888) are discussed in Chapter Two. Chapter Three examines Eduard Albert's *Die Frauen und das Studium der Medizin* (1895), Chapter Four analyzes Max Runge's *Das Weib in seiner geschlechtlichen Eigenart* (1897), and Chapter Five focuses on Paul Julius Möbius' *Über den physiologischen Schwachsinn des Weibes* (1901). As indicated by the titles listed here in chronological order, the focus of these (pseudo) scientific explorations changes over the years. The first three texts seem to be concerned specifically with women and medical education; the latter two attempt to create a new kind of female psychology. Although all these texts contain both elements, it is important to acknowledge that each of them also accentuates a different aspect of the so-called female nature: the anatomical structure of the whole body and brain, the reproductive organs, and female physiological functions. These five treatises are by no means the only texts opposing or even warning about admission of women to medical schools, but these are the texts that elicited the most responses from contemporary women.[19]

In my discussion of these (pseudo) scientific texts and responses they generated I chose a thematic focus for each of the five chapters. In Chapter One, I introduce the main concepts pertaining to the question of higher, especially medical, education for women in the second half of the nineteenth century that will be developed in the course of this book. In particular, I show how this question relates to the broader agenda of gender politics. I demonstrate that the public debate surrounding the issue was not concerned with education as such, but rather focused on the female body and sexuality. I also provide a historical overview of the struggle for women's admission to medical schools in Germany and Austria within a broader European context, and I present early feminists' critical analyses of the hostile German and Austrian positions. In Chapter Two, I introduce the first stage of the debate regarding women's admission to medical schools that was focused on the female brain. I demonstrate how, by responding to texts on the brain structure and anatomical differences between males and females, many of the progressive writers questioned the validity of a worldview based on the dichotomy of reason and emotion. In addition, I examine how the categories of

19 For more titles, see Sveistrup and Zahn-Harnack 467-79.

class and gender intersected in this debate and discuss a connection between (pseudo) scientific pamphlets and political decisions. In Chapter Three, I examine the distinction between the public and private spaces as a gender-constitutive characteristic. In addition, I argue that the space itself is gendered. I show how the categories of gender (male/female), space (public/private), and class (bourgeois/working-class) intersect with each other creating multiple female gender types. In this context, a new identity emerges: the female student. The public space of the university becomes a site of the negotiation of this new identity. I also demonstrate that middle-class women's confinement to the private realm simultaneously created epistemological boundaries. By transgressing these boundaries, middle-class women strove to destabilize the prevailing notion of femininity. Finally, I discuss the notion of the female body as an object of aesthetic and sensual pleasure. The main focus of Chapter Four is the process of knowledge production and dissemination regarding the female body and its reproductive sexuality by mainstream scientists, as well as the feminist intervention in this process. Specifically, I investigate the means by which this knowledge was produced and the different ways by which it was acquired. I juxtapose the medical knowledge monopolized by male physicians to women's knowledge of their own bodies as thematized in the feminist press of the time. In addition, this chapter investigates intersections of popular science, early feminist thought, and the politics of reproduction in the context of women's struggle for academic education. In Chapter Five, I demonstrate that the (pseudo) scientific texts about femininity can be read as cultural manifestos aimed at reversing emancipatory tendencies of modernity. In addition, I argue that they can be situated in a framework of what I refer to as the pornographic imagination. I also show how the discussion about "female nature" is embedded in concepts of nature and culture. Finally, I provide the perspectives of many nineteenth-century middle-class women on the shift in the popular understanding of femininity that took place as a result of women's struggle for admission to higher education. Each chapter centers on a specific text (or texts) written by opponents to women's medical education and on a specific set of themes. I chose the particular themes for each chapter based on what I believe was the most important issue addressed by intellectuals and activists responding to these texts.

1 The Struggle for Women's Admission to Medical Schools: Politics of the Female Body

Perhaps a future generation will read with astonishment of the old dispute about the question of 'female physicians,' and scarcely believe that there has ever been such a dispute.

Elizabeth Garrett-Anderson[20]

1.1 Introduction: Historical Overview

Eliza Ichenhaeuser, an active supporter of female academic education at the end of the nineteenth century, pointed out that by 1897 women's struggle for freedom, rooted in a general feeling of social injustice and inequality, had transformed itself into a well-organized movement with concrete demands and tangible plans for ending discrimination against women. She identified four main arenas in which women demanded equality: economy, law, education, and politics.[21] According to Ichenhaeuser, economic emancipation had received the most social approval due to alarming statistics documenting the constantly growing number of single women without the means to live. Women's equality before the law, although recognized as a social necessity, had received inadequate social support. Ichenhaeuser saw the fear that male privileges would subsequently be limited as the main cause of the relatively low social support for ending discrimination against women before the law. Finally, Ichenhaeuser argued, women's intellectual and political emancipation evoked rather negative feelings in German society and was perceived as questionable and even dangerous (*Ausnahmestellung* 3-5). However, Ichenhaeuser recognized that intellectual emancipation was the basis for equality in all other fields. She argued that higher education was necessary for women to gain access to liberal professions and become physicians, lawyers, and teachers. It was crucial to establish female representation in fields that influenced the understanding of gender differences, created laws, and regulated social interactions among and between genders because men usually represented only male and not female interests:

20 Qtd. in the 1890 English edition of Helene Lange, *Higher Education of Women in Europe* 54.

21 Other activists of the women's movement identified slightly different fields of the desired emancipation. Therese Schlesinger, for example, advocated "ökonomische, politische, intellektuelle und sexuelle Emanzipation" (Bandhauer-Schöffmann 60-61).

> [E]s [ist] für die gesammte Frauenwelt ein schreiendes Bedürfnis [...], dass ihre starkgeistigen, bedeutenden Schwestern sich voll und ganz entwickeln können zu Nutz und Frommen des ganzen Geschlechts. Die Frauen brauchen weibliche Ärzte, nicht allein um ihre Krankheiten zu heilen, sondern auch um ihr Bestes, ihre Keuschheit zu hüten, sie brauchen weibliche Juristen, die an der Gesetzgebung, die die Frau betrifft, mitarbeiten müssen, sie brauchen akademisch gebildete, weibliche Lehrer, die den Mädchen-Unterricht reformieren müssen, kurzum, sie brauchen auf allen Gebieten führende Geister *ihres* Geschlechts. (Ichenhaeuser, *Ausnahmestellung* 20-21)

However, access to education and liberal professions was only one side of women's intellectual emancipation. The other aspect, not addressed by Ichenhaeuser, was the development of a new self-understanding by women that would be based on their own needs and on their own awareness. Both processes were interdependent and required a re-definition of gender roles. Ute Frevert, writing in 1988, argued that precisely the self-understanding of middle-class women as unequal to men was the biggest obstacle on the road to emancipation. She wrote: "Mächtiger noch als die äußeren Widerstände, denen Frauen in der staatlichen Bürokratie, in den bürgerlichen Parteien oder in der eigenen Familie begegneten, waren oft ihre inneren Barrieren gegen den Gedanken einer radikalen Gleichheit männlicher und weiblicher Lebensmodelle" (Frevert 18). Therefore, the development of a new self-perception by women was crucial to any possibility of change of the existing views of femininity.

Women's growing awareness of their underprivileged position in society sparked the desire for a better education. Consequently, the second half of the nineteenth century was clearly marked by a progressive intensification of women's efforts to gain access to higher education.[22] Since barring women from universities

22 Weiershausen provides in her book a detailed bibliography of predominantly German publications dealing with the sociohistorical background of the struggle for the admission of women to higher education: scholarly literature dealing with specific universities or selected academic disciplines (especially medicine); comparative works exploring developments of higher education for women specifically in Germany, Austria, and Switzerland or including other countries; and biographies and autobiographies of first female students (20-22). In addition to the bibliography included by Weiershausen, the following publications provide a good analysis of the relevant sociohistorical context: Heindl, Waltraud and Marina Tichy, eds. *"Durch Erkenntnis zu Freiheit und Glück..." Frauen an der Universität Wien (ab 1897).* Wien: Universitätsverlag, 1990; Brinkschulte, Eva, ed. *Weibliche Ärzte. Die Durchsetzung des Berufsbildes in Deutschland,* Berlin: Edition Hentrich und bei dem Institut für Geschichte der Medizin der Freien Universität Berlin, 1993; Ziegeler, Beate. *Weibliche Ärzte und Krankenkassen. Anfänge ärztlicher Berufstätigkeit von Frauen in Berlin 1893-1935.* Weinheim: Deutscher Studien Verlag, 1993; Koerner, Marianne. *Auf fremdem Terrain. Studien- und Alltagserfahrungen von Studentinnen 1900 bis 1918.* Bonn: Didot-Verlag Sabine Dörrich, 1997. Mazón provides a helpful overview of the contemporary research approaches to issue of higher education of women in the nineteenth century (12-15). She

was based on a general exclusion of women from the public sphere and on rigid sex-specific norms of behavior underlying this exclusion, supporters of female education demanded a re-evaluation of strictly defined gender roles[23] by questioning prevailing conceptions of femininity. Consequently, at the core of the discussion regarding admission of women to higher education that dominated public life at the end of the nineteenth century was the normative discourse on the female body and sexuality.

Among all academic disciplines being discussed as potentially open to women, medicine created the greatest controversies, drawing substantial public attention as a result.[24] On the one hand, the initial response of the majority of medical doctors and professors to the first women attempting to gain admission to medical schools was one of categorical rejection. Professors sitting on the admissions boards refused to accept female students to medical schools in most European countries, employing as one of the main arguments the inherent intellectual inferiority that made it impossible for women to think rationally and to understand abstract concepts.[25] Although initially the idea of granting women regular admission to a university was received negatively among faculty members in all academic disciplines throughout Europe, doctors and professors of medicine put up the most obstinate resistance.[26] While discussing female education, Helene Lange pointed out that even in England, a country that was relatively open to women's academic demands, the profession of a physician was perceived as part of an exclusively male domain. She wrote: "Nur in einem Fache war auch in England ein ernstlicher Kampf gegen Vorurteile und – Brotneid zu kämpfen: in der Medizin" (*Frauenbildung* 29). On the other hand, medicine as a profession was especially appealing to women from a pragmatic as well as a historically logical standpoint because women were traditionally in a position to care for and to nurture those who were sick. In addition to giving women job opportunities and financial independence, it provided a professional application of characteristics believed to be a well-defined part of female nature such as tenderness, caring for

---

divides the scholarship into the following categories: (1) "documentary histories of women at individual universities," (2) "works by historians of Germany that place women's education in a larger interpretive framework," and (3) "diverse feminist approaches" (12). See also Mazón's discussion of arguments made by James Albisetti, Claudia Huerkamp, Londa Schiebinger, Edith Glaser (12-13) and footnotes 42, 43, and 44 (231-232).

23 Mazón also uses the phrase "strictly defined gender roles" (2). She also writes: "The starting point for these constraints was the narrow definition of both male and female roles. While woman's destiny confines her to the home, a man's suited him for a more active role outside of the family" (49).

24 See also Heindl, "Zur Entwicklung des Frauenstudiums in Österreich" 22; Tichy, "Die geschlechtliche Un-Ordnung" 28-29.

25 See, for example, the arguments made by Siegfried Placzek (qtd. in Schmersahl 306-307).

26 See also Tichy, "Die geschlechtliche Un-Ordnung" 28-29; Heindl, "Zur Entwicklung des Frauenstudiums in Österreich" 22; Brinkschulte, "Dr. med. Maria Daelen" 5; Glaser, "Die erste Studentinnengeneration" 318.

others, empathy, and compassion.[27] Moreover, supporters of women's medical education often referred to the centuries-old practice of female healers and midwives.[28] Hedwig Dohm, for instance, in her book *Die wissenschaftliche Emanzipation der Frau*, provided a detailed and well-researched history of female healers throughout the ages (101-16). She claimed that obstetrics had always been perceived as a naturally female domain and that in some countries male physicians were even prohibited from performing gynecological procedures (*Emancipation* 110). Dohm pointed out that it was only due to the lack of female participation in the legislative process that men started dominating the field of obstetrics.

> Wie geschah es nun, daß die Männer einen Zweig der Heilkunde an sich reißen konnten, von dem Gesetz, Kirche und Schamhaftigkeit in früheren Jahrhunderten sie fern gehalten hatte? Sehr einfach. Die Willkür der Gesetzgebung, an welcher Frauen keinen Antheil hatten, verbot eines Tages der Frau das Studium und die Ausübung der Medizin. Der Gesetzgeber rief den Geburtshelfer ins Leben und unterdrückte trotz Vernunft, Schamhaftigkeit und individueller Freiheit das gemeinsame Recht. (*Emanzipation* 112)

It is not surprising that such views created a tremendous amount of controversy. Opinions such as Dohm's not only threatened to undermine male dominance in the medical profession, but also the status quo of a patriarchal society.

Given that medical discourse played a major role in defining biological differences between the sexes and in determining gender roles in society, the discussion surrounding the admission of women to medical schools necessarily generated a debate about female nature.[29] However, it is important to clarify that scientific explorations of femininity in the nineteenth century often only mirrored and justified the deeply rooted popular understanding of gender differences, based on the perception of a dichotomy between mind and body, culture and nature, good and evil, a dichotomy that attributed mind, culture, and good to men and body, nature, and evil to women.[30] While men were believed to be able to transcend bodily limitations, being a woman meant being defined by sexuality and being limited to physiological functions alone.

---

27 See also Rohner 11; Burchardt 14; Twellmann qtd. in Weiershausen 37-38; Schmersahl 303; Mazón 94.

28 See also Rohner 9-10.

29 Weiershausen points out that one of the main reasons for the controversies surrounding medical education for women was "die Verknüpfung mit dem Körper- und Sexualdiskurs sowie durch die spezielle Rolle der Medizin für den Geschlechterdiskurs der Zeit" (38). In this context, Weiershausen also refers to Claudia Honegger's research (38-39).

30 Schmersahl demonstrated a close relationship between medical theories and popular perception of gender differences. She emphasized, for example, "[d]ie direkte Abhängigkeit medizinischer Krankheits- und Gesundheitskonzeptionen von den zeitgenössischen Vorstellungen über das Geschlechterverhältnis" (1).

At the same time, as many women started demanding equal rights by explicitly questioning the prevalent notion of femininity, scientists attempted to justify the imposition of even stricter gender boundaries between men and women, utilizing deterministic biological arguments, particularly in relation to reproductive functions.[31] Hence, the discussion surrounding the entrance of women into the medical field clearly illuminates gender politics at the end of the nineteenth century. It also reflects the painful process of changing social consciousness regarding the notion of femininity.

In the European context, Germany and Austria were not among the pioneers of female medical education. On the contrary, both countries struggled for a long time before they embraced this idea. Although a few women were able to attend academic lectures as *Gasthörerinnen* in Germany and Austria at selected universities before 1900,[32] laws sanctioning the admission of female students as a regular practice were not passed until much later.[33] These laws were subject to the jurisdiction of each state and were ratified in each state at a different time "between 1900 and 1909" (Mazón 10; 137) and in many cases referred to specific fields and not to all academic disciplines. The last four German states to sanction women's entrance to the academic field were Prussia (1908), Alsace-Lorraine (1908), Hessen (1908), and Mecklenburg, which issued a law to this effect in 1909 (Burchardt 16; Weiershausen 9; Mazón 10).[34] Women had been granted admission privileges much earlier in some countries, although in the United States, England, and Russia separate academic departments for women were created. The United States admitted women in 1850/56, France in 1863, Switzerland/Zurich in 1865, Sweden in 1870, England and Russia in 1872, Denmark in 1875, Italy in 1876, Holland in 1878, Norway in 1882, and Belgium in 1883 (Rohner 90).[35] The

---

31 Weiershausen uses a similar argument: "Die konkrete Debatte um die Zulassung von Frauen zum Medizinstudium lieferte [...] Beispiele für den Umgang mit Geschlechtsdefinitionen, die dem Ausschluß von Frauen dienten" (48). Schmersahl also argued that: "Je weniger die soziale Realität dem Postulat der Geschlechterpolarität entsprach, umso lauter klagten die Mediziner die Einhaltung der Geschlechterrollen ein" (310).

32 See also Mazón 10.

33 For a detailed discussion of the legislation and timeline of women's admission to the universities in Austria (particularly in Vienna) see Heindl, "Zur Entwicklung des Frauenstudiums in Österreich" 17-26; Bandhauer-Schöffmann 49-78; Tuma 79-92; Wytek 153-85. For a timeline of women's admission to the universities and legislation regarding the issue of medical education for women in Germany see Burchardt 16; 19; Brinkschulte 22-23; Glaser, "Die erste Studentinnengemeration" 310 and footnotes (596-97); Mazón 115-151.

34 For a detailed discussion of the positions and legislations of specific German states up to 1903 see Ichenhaeuser, "Die Frauenstudienfrage in Deutschland" 1052-58. See also Mazón 137-144.

35 See also Heindl, "Zur Entwicklung des Frauenstudiums" 17; Lange, *Frauenbildung* 30-30, 76-77; Ichenhaeuser, "Ausnahmestellung" 43-44; Burchardt 13, 18; Brinkschulte, *Weibliche Ärzte* 22; Schmersahl 304. Since in some cases regulation of the issue of women's admission was left to the authorities of a particular university or even to the specific professors, and in others it was based on general legislation, it is difficult to provide specific dates of general

practice of allowing women to participate in higher education started in most of the countries as an exception made for selected individuals and usually became a regular practice shortly thereafter. Switzerland, one of the first countries to grant women access to higher education, followed this characteristic path. In 1864 and 1865, two Russian women, Maria Kniaschnina and Nadescha Suslowa, enrolled at the university in Zurich (Rohner 12).[36] This event led women from other European countries that did not allow them access to higher education to apply to the medical school in Zurich (Rohner 12). Consequently, in the following months, the admission of women became a regular practice at the university in Zurich, causing numerous protests, especially in Austria and Germany (Rohner 13). The decision of the academic authorities in Zurich obviously undermined popularly held convictions about a female's inability to study subjects such as medicine (Rohner 13). Despite the fact that Zurich provided tangible proof that women were capable of rational and abstract thinking, many scientists decided to see the intellect of these women as a pathological manifestation[37] rather than as an integral part of femininity and refused to reconsider the so-called characteristics of female nature. Auguste Forel, a Swiss professor of medicine and proponent of female education, responded to the protests by advocating a trial method:[38]

> Entweder sind die Frauen zum Hochschulstudium befähigt, dann wäre es feige und brutal – ein Abusus roher Kraft, es ihnen etwa aus Konkurrenzangst zu verwehren. Oder sie sind dazu nicht befähigt – dann werden sie schon von selber im Kampf für die Existenz allmählich unterliegen und man hat ebenfalls keinen Grund, ihnen den Versuch zu verwehren. (qtd. in Rohner 13)

Most of the German and Austrian universities rejected this progressive attitude,[39] at least during the first thirty years after the Swiss precedent. The authorities, faculty members, and scientists refused to question the validity of arguments based on the notion of inborn and unchangeable gender characteristics that condemned

---

admission of women to universities throughout Europe. There is also no consensus in the literature regarding dates of opening universities to women.

36 See also Weiershausen 13.

37 Tichy uses the expression "[d]ie Verpathologisierung weiblicher Intellektualität" ("Die geschlechtliche Un-Ordnung" 40). Schmersahl argues: "Einer Frau, die sich nicht an die geschlechtlichen Schranken hielt, drohte die Pathologisierung" (104). See also Schmersahl 103-105.

38 Many female activists advocated a similar trial method, see Bandhauer-Schöffmann 63-64.

39 See also Rohner 13; 65; Schmersahl 307-308. Schmersahl writes: "Viele deutsche Ärzte beharrten trotz oder wegen der inzwischen jahrezehntelangen positiven Erfahrungen im Ausland mit Ärztinnen umso mehr auf ihrer misogynen und antiemanzipatorischen Haltung. Die auch in deutschen Fachzeitschriften teilweise veröffentlichten Artikel, in denen die zumeist ausländische Verfasser für die Öffnung der deutschen medizinischen Fakultäten für Frauen plädierten, konnten die Mehrheit der deutschen Ärzte nicht umstimmen" (307).

women to inevitable failure in any intellectual endeavors. The opposition to Zurich's admission of women was based on its perceived (but not articulated) potential as a threat to other universities. If others followed Zurich's example, the position of all opponents of female higher education would be weakened. In truth, the fears of the opponents were well founded. The precedent set by the university in Zurich enabled advocates of female education to demand the same right for women elsewhere.

The rapidly growing number of female medical students throughout Europe illustrates the progressive change in attitudes towards the admission of women to medical schools. At the same time, authorities and faculty members at German and Austrian universities continued to work against the admission of female students. *Die Versammlung Deutscher Naturforscher und Ärzte* declared officially in 1879 that it would not accept women's presence at universities under any circumstances (Brinkschulte, *Weibliche Ärzte* 22). This decision of German scientists and doctors was announced after many women had already been admitted to medical schools in several European countries. Physicians and academics in Germany evidently felt threatened by the increasing support for female education throughout Europe and tried to respond with organized resistance. At the same time, however, more proponents of female education started emerging among academics and intellectuals in Germany and Austria; for example, a contemporary historian Waltraud Heindl mentions that Edmund Bernatzik, an Austrian law professor, condemned the restrictions placed on women as unconstitutional, pointing to the eighteenth paragraph of the constitution: "Es steht jedermann frei, seinen Beruf zu wählen und sich für denselben auszubilden, wie und wo er will" (qtd. in Heindl, "Zur Entwicklung des Frauenstudiums" 20).[40]

In spite of the growing number of supporters of female medical education in Austria and Germany, the first female students in these countries were officially admitted to medical schools approximately thirty-six years after women were able to study in Zurich. In this struggle, the following four factors played a major role in the enforcement of female medical education in Austria and Germany: the long-time intervention of various women's organizations at state and university levels;[41] the dissemination of progressive ideas through the journals of the women's movement, such as *Die Frau*, *Die Frauenbewegung*, and *Dokumente der Frauen/ Frauen-Rundschau*; the activism of dedicated individual proponents of female education; and the fact that, by the end of the nineteenth century, the universities

40 See also Bandhauer-Schöffmann 67.

41 See also Heindl and Tichy, "Einleitung" 9; Glaser, "Die erste Studentinnengeneration" 310; Brinkschulte, *Weibliche Ärzte* 22. For the discussion of the intervention of Austrian women's organisatioins see Bandauer-Schöffmann 49-78. For the discussion of the intervention of German women's organisations see Glaser, "Die erste Studentinnengeneration" 311-18. Mazón, however, argues that "[g]overnments never acted on the [...] petitions" submitted by the advocates of higher education for women (71). See also Mazón 60 and footnote 23 (242).

in many European countries had already admitted women to medical schools.[42] In addition to these factors, Heindl speaks of a demographic development that supported the struggle of the women's movement: at a time when there were more women than men, the traditional gender roles could be easily undermined because not all women could count on marriage as the financial basis of their existence ("Zur Entwicklung des Frauenstudiums in Österreich" 22).[43] Furthermore, the unstable economic situation created an environment susceptible to the demands of higher education for women, since many bourgeois wives and daughters were forced to search for additional sources of income to help sustain their families.[44] In particular, the *Allgemeine Deutsche Frauenverein* (ADF)[45] and the *Allgemeine Österreichische Frauenverein* (AÖF) perceived the unrestricted access to education, as well as the right to work for bourgeois women, as the main goals of their political and social struggle. Louise Otto Peters, the founder of ADF, summarized the objectives of the women's movement as follows: "die erhöhte Bildung des weiblichen Geschlechts und die Befreiung der weiblichen Arbeit von allen ihrer Entfaltung entgegenstehenden Hindernissen" (qtd. in Glaser, "Die erste Studentinnengeneration" 311). Similarly, the AÖF chose the following motto for its agitation: "Durch Erkenntnis zu Freiheit und Glück" (Heindl and Tichy, "Einleitung" 9). In the decade between 1889 and 1899, organizations of the women's movement issued numerous petitions to the German and Austrian parliaments demanding the admission of women to higher education and the abolition of restrictions placed on middle-class women regarding professional work.[46]

Yet women aspiring to medical education and to financial independence had to overcome more obstacles than just obtaining permission to attend lectures and seminars. In the first place, they had to attain a level of education corresponding to the requirements of the universities. For this reason, appropriate secondary schools had to be established. These schools would prepare girls to take the final examinations (*Abitur/Matura*) and to obtain a secondary school certificate

42 See also Glaser, "Sind Frauen studierfähig?" 306. Mazón referrs to an argument made by James Albisetti that "German officials were finally pushed to admit women to medical certification for fear of appearing retrograde compared to other countries" (Mazón 13-14).

43 See also Weiershausen 20; Mazón 51-52.

44 Heindl, "Zur Entwicklung des Frauenstudiums" 22-23; Tichy, "Die geschlechtliche Un-Ordnung" 27-28; Glaser, "Die erste Studentinnengeneration" 313.

45 For a discussion of ADF's efforts to grant women access to higher education see Mazón 58-63.

46 Bandahauer-Schöffmann 49-78; Brinkschulte, *Weibliche Ärzte* (timeline) 22; Glaser, "Die erste Studentinnengeneration" 311-18. Mazón focuses on the efforts of ADF that, according to her, "embarked on an active petition campaign on behalf of female higher education" between 1888 and 1902 (59). She also claims that "[t]he years from 1887 to 1894 saw the greatest number of petitions submitted to the *Reichstag*, state legislatures, and state education ministers on behalf of the *Frauenstudium*" (Mazón 79).

enabling their admission to the universities.[47] The *Abitur/Matura* requirement applied also to men, but unlike high schools for boys, schools for girls did not prepare girls for this kind of examination. Mazón argues that "requiring female applicants to take this exam served to divert the onslaught of women students officials had feared" (5). However, the *Abitur/Matura* requirement is understandable from the point of view of university authorities concerned with the standards of higher education (Mazón 2). In Germany, Helene Lange made a breakthrough in 1889 by establishing courses in Berlin *(Realkurse für Frauen)* that prepared women for the *Abitur* and for university education.[48] In Austria, where until 1903 there was only one *Mädchengymnasium* comparable to the male educational institutions, Marianne Hainisch campaigned for seconday schools for girls.[49] As Mazón points out, before women were officially admitted to universities (in each state at a different time "between 1900 and 1909") and hence allowed to enroll as regular students, the only option they had was to audit classes (10; 117; 137). Although very few women audited classes in Germany before 1870, in the late 1870s and in the 1880s women were banned from auditing classes at almost all universities in Germany (Mazón 10; 119). This ban was lifted in the 1890s (Mazón 10; 119). Depending on the particular university, women were allowed to audit only selected courses and had to obtain permission from university authorities, from the individual professor, and in many cases also from the state minister of education (Mazón 122; Ichenhaeuser, *Ausnahmestellung* 44-45). Further restrictions were placed on women who managed to finish a course of studies because they could not receive a degree without, again, petitioning to various authorities (Mazón 107). Medical education was a special case because it required extensive practical experience. In 1899 women were given permission to take the medical state certification exam (Staatsexamen),[50] but beforehand they were unable to work in hospitals or to establish private practices. In addition, women could rarely find a doctor who would accept females as assistants or trainees in a hospital. Beate Ziegler points to these limited opportunities to gain experience necessary in the medical profession; for example, in the 1890s there was only one German physician who employed female assistants (*Weibliche Ärzte* 11).[51] Women were confronted by a similar situation in Austria, where directors in the Viennese hospitals refused to employ women as well (Ziegler, *Weibliche Ärzte* 12). Women who decided to graduate abroad still had to overcome various obstacles if they

---

47 For a brief discussion of education for girls see Mazón 51-52. For a discussion of different secondary school models see Mazón 62-63; 70-73; 79-80.

48 Burchardt 12; Bäumer, "Das Mädchenbildung" 123; Heinsohn 151; Ziegeler, *Weibliche Ärzte* 26. See also Mazón 78-80. For a detailed discussion of secondary schools preparing girls for higher education in Germany see Burchardt 12; Bäumer, "Die Mädchenbildung" 123-27; Heinsohn 149-54.

49 Heindl, "Zur Entwicklung des Frauenstudiums" 23-24; Bandauer-Schöffmann 51; 54.

50 Burchardt 16; Schmersahl 305; Mazon 112.

51 For a detailed discussion of this issue see Ziegeler, *Weibliche Ärzte* 11-13.

wanted to work as physicians in Germany and Austria. Most problematic was the refusal to recognize medical degrees from universities abroad and the ruling that prohibited women educated in a foreign country to use the title "doctor."[52] This law was not overruled in Austria until 1896 and in Germany until 1899 when women were able to obtain the title through the medical state certification exam.[53] In other words, until the early twentieth century women were prohibited from practicing the medical profession in Austria and Germany by all possible legal and illegal means, even though many had received the proper education and training.[54]

1.2 Position on Female Education Peculiar to Germany and Austria

By 1896, women had been granted full access to higher education, including medical schools, in almost all European countries with the exception of Austria and Germany. In her book entitled *Die Ausnahmestellung Deutschlands in Sachen Frauenstudium* (1898), Eliza Ichenhaeuser portrays this situation as follows:

> In der ganzen civilisierten Welt sind den Frauen die Universitäten offen. [...] Deutschland und Österreich allein haben sich den Ruhm vorbehalten, die Veste des Vorurtheils am längsten vertheidigt zu haben, sogar Ungarn hat den Frauen im vorigen Jahre [1896] die Zulassung ertheilt, aber Oesterreich begnügte sich mit der Nostrifikation der im Ausland studiert habenden Aerztinnen, trotzdem gerade Oesterreich Aerztinnen in seinen Okkupationsländern nothwendig braucht, und Deutschland verharrt noch ganz auf dem alten Standpunkt. (43-44)

At the end of the nineteenth century, many activists and intellectuals reflected on the hostile position of Germany and Austria regarding education for women, especially in the medical field. In their writings, they specifically emphasized the open opposition as well as passive indifference of influential individuals and members of the medical profession that interfered with and sabotaged women's demands. The stark differences distinguishing Austria/Germany from elsewhere in Europe become evident in the specific examples provided by these activists. Lina Morgenstern, for instance, speaks of the support for female medical education in Russia. Not only had the Russian government established numerous medical schools for women and employed many female physicians, but also Russian scientists had actively supported women in their struggle. During the first official meeting of Russian scientists and physicians in Odessa in 1883, the participating

---

52 Bandhauer-Schöffmann 63; Burchardt 15; Bornemann 29; Hoesch 48; Ziegeler, *Weibliche Ärzte* 15; 67. For a detailed discussion of the legal matters see Ziegeler, *Weibliche Ärzte* 15-27.

53 Burchardt 16; Bandhauer-Schöffmann 64.

54 See also Burchardt 16-17.

men encouraged female involvement and even chose women as chairs of many sessions and divisions ("Vorsitzende einzelner Abteilungen") (Morgenstern 9). Morgenstern quotes Professor Sklifassowski, one of the participants of the Odessa meeting:

> Wir haben die Frau in den Räumen der Universität kennen gelernt, als Kreisarzt auf dem Lande gesehen; wir haben sie als Arzt auf den Schlachtfeldern bewundert und überall hat sie sich unsere Sympathien erworben und sich würdig gezeigt, auf einer Stufe mit den Männern zu stehen. (Morgenstern 10)

This passage exemplifies the sharp divergence of the general Russian and German positions. As already noted, in Germany only four years earlier, in 1879, members of *Die Versammlung Deutscher Naturforscher und Ärzte* had refused categorically to accept women's presence in medical schools and were still putting up fierce resistance. Like Russia, England provided a positive example. Helene Lange refers to the support of English authorities for female medical education. She mentions a speech by Lord Granville, chancellor of the University of London, of June 29, 1888, in which he congratulated female medical students of England for their courage, hard work, and success. Further, Lord Granville expressed his support for women who decided to pursue medical careers (*Frauenbildung* 40-42). Lange points out that, at the same time, Prussian parliamentarians responsible for reviewing the question of female education tabled the issue by concluding "Die Welt werde nicht untergehen, wenn die Frauen noch warteten" (*Frauenbildung* 42). Mathilde Weber and Lina Morgenstern draw attention to the fact that the Queen of Italy and the Queen of Romania nominated female medical doctors to be their personal physicians (Weber 51; Morgenstern 15). By doing so, both queens made a statement "daß sie es für notwendig and segensvoll halten, wenn Frauen sich dem medizinischen Berufe zuwenden" (Morgenstern 15).

The question of why the German situation was so abnormal permeates all these examples. Lange attempted to provide an answer by examining three possible causes: external adverse circumstances, men's unwillingness to aid the cause, and women's indifference.[55] She analyzed the German situation and concluded that the external circumstances in Germany were not different from those in other European countries in regard to potential female education. The possibility of some men losing jobs and women taking their place existed everywhere. Consequently, fear of competition could not be solely a German phenomenon. Further, the structure and workings of universities were similar everywhere in Europe. If women's presence in the public space of academia did not harm anybody in any way in Europe or North America, it would most likely

55 "Adverse Circumstances," "Men's Unwillingness to aid the Cause," and "Women's Indifference" are used as chapter headings by the translator of the English edition of Lange's book, *Higher Education of Women in Europe*, L.R. Klemm in the "contents" section.

not have had a negative influence in Germany either. In addition, Germany was not a poor country; it had the necessary means to support female education financially. In short, according to Lange, external circumstances were not responsible for the failure to grant women admission to universities in Germany (*Frauenbildung* 97-101).

Two remaining causes seem to offer an answer to the inquiries regarding the peculiarity of the German and Austrian situations. According to Lange, male unwillingness to aid the cause of women's admission to medical schools and female indifference to the movement were the main reasons for the fruitless struggle in Germany. In addition to openly opposing female education out of a sense of competition, fear, intellectual arrogance, and misogyny, most men did not support the cause for two main reasons: ignorance of and/or indifference toward the situation of women. Lange writes: "Sie [die Männer] haben über die Frauenfrage nie nachgedacht. Sie kennen die Notlage nicht, die sie geschaffen [haben]" (*Frauenbildung* 102). She points out that in Germany the most common male response to women's demands regarding higher education was mockery. However, she insists that such a response could only arise from unawareness and lack of knowledge of the subject of women's struggle. Quoting a passage from the journal *Familie und Individuum* she elaborates on this issue:

> Und in der That kann der Spott auf diesem Gebiete keinen anderen Ursprung, als den der vollständigen Unkenntnis haben. Jeder Mann, und hätte er auch nur ein halbes Gewissen, müßte erschrecken, wenn man ihn durch das thatsächliche Elend, dem die Frauenbewegung entsprungen, überzeugte, daß er auf Kosten dieses Elends seinen Witz übt, daß er mit diesem Spott, den er so siegesgewiß führt, tausend Möglichkeiten tötete, die dem hungernden Brot, dem Unglücklichen Glück, ja dem auf ehrlosen Wegen Wandelnden die Ehre hätten retten können. (*Frauenbildung* 103)

In reference to the notion of male ignorance of the issue, Lange blames German women who do not inform men about the hardships of female existence. In other words, female indifference to the women's movement for admission to medical schools damaged the cause. According to Lange, women remained too passive and did not attempt to gain male support for their cause. Similarly, Weber points the finger at the majority of German women who, unlike women in other countries, did not participate actively in the struggle. According to her, German women tended to demonstrate passivity and showed a lack of interest in female education (Weber 23). Only a combined effort of all German women could grant a successful outcome:

> Gewiß würden das Vorurteil und der Widerstand dagegen [gegen weibliche Ärzte] leichter gebrochen, wenn alle Mütter in gemein-

> samer Übereinstimmung erklären würden: "Nachdem wir in anderen Ländern treffliche weibliche Ärzte wirken sehen, wünschen auch wir unseren Töchtern und uns selbst die Seelenqual und das Erröten zu ersparen, über alle diese Krankheitssymptome mit einem Manne zu verhandeln." (Weber 23-24)

In addition to male ignorance and female passivity, many supporters of women's education also pointed to a third factor: the "German tendency" to discuss an issue theoretically instead of relying on empirical experiment. According to these critics, Germany, as the homeland of philosophers and thinkers, had a tendency toward theoretical speculation. It seemed to constitute one of the German national characteristics and affected the struggle for women's education in a negative way. Sidonie Binder writes: "Fast in der ganzen Welt giebt es weibliche Aerzte. [...] Aber im Lande der Theorie, in Deutschland, erklären viele trotzdem die Sache heute noch überhaupt für existenzunmöglich" (18). Likewise, Weber calls attention to the fact that almost all European countries had tried empirically "was wir [Deutsche] noch theoretisch bekämpfen" (29). Both Weber and Morgenstern refer to Dr. Hause and his "Brief an eine Mutter"[56] in which he wrote: "Wir Deutsche haben die Gewohnheit, über Probleme zu klügeln und zu philosophieren, über die Möglichkeit der Ausführung und den Wert oder Unwert einer Sache zu tifteln und zu streiten, und ehe wir einig geworden, haben bereits die anderen Nationen das Beste davon weggenommen" (Weber 45; Morgenstern 15).

Active opponents of female education did not constitute a coherent social group. According to Weber, who attempted to discover who these people were and why they resisted women's entrance into medical schools, there were three major groups of opponents. The first group included all those who were enslaved by social traditions and habits ("diejenigen, welche sich schwer losmachen aus den Banden des Allgewohnten und Hergebrachten") (Weber 19). They feared negative social changes and potential obliteration of the established social order. Legislative authorities, such as members of parliament and ministries constituted the second group. In spite of the positive reactions of some individuals, these authorities on the whole sabotaged women's demand for educational equality by abdicating responsibility:

> [D]ie Minister der einzelnen Länder sagten: das sei Sache des Reichs und des Bundesrates; dort aber wurde man berichtet, das sei Sache der einzelnen Landtage, und von hier schickte man uns wieder an den Reichstag; derselbe erklärte trotz der warmen Fürsprache einzelner Mitglieder des hohen Hauses in der Sitzung vom 11. März 1891, er sei nicht kompetent, und ging zur Tagesordnung über. (Weber 20)

56 They do not provide any further information about the text or its author. Morgenstern refers to "Briefe an eine Mutter" (15) and Weber to "Brief an eine Mutter"(45).

The third group consisted of physicians and professors of medicine who took the most active stance on the issue, since they felt directly affected by women's demands. Although some of them seemed to be genuinely worried about female health, most were motivated by fear of competition in the job market and an intellectual arrogance ("aus geistigem Hochmut") that dreaded the thought of inferior creatures, women, wanting to succeed in a "male" profession (Weber 20).

Active supporters of female entrance into academia, on the other hand, were a socially coherent group, mainly middle-class progressive and educated women.[57] Of course, there were also male supporters of women's education, but they were a minority and in general not as vocal and demanding as women. On petitions submitted to the German parliament the majority of signatures were those of women. In 1889, Lange wrote: "Versuche, auch in Deutschland den Frauen den Zugang zu den Universitäten zu verschaffen, sind in den letzten Jahrzehnten vielfach gemacht worden, wenn auch nur von ihrem eigenen Geschlecht. Einzelne Professoren sind auch in Deutschland der Sache freundlich gesinnt, ohne sich aber zum Vorkämpfer der Frauen aufzuwerfen" (*Frauenbildung* 80). However, as I will demonstrate in the following chapters, the number of active supporters increased over time. Gradually, the issue of female education (especially medical) elicited more and more positive responses in Germany and Austria.

Of course, there is no simple explanation of the very peculiar German and Austrian positions on the issue of higher education for women. The responses by Lange, Binder, Weber, and Morgenstern provided valuable insights and revealed nineteenth-century perspectives on the subject. Their explanations, however, do not seem to give a complete answer. Summarizing approaches and findings of contemporary scholarship, Mazón points out that the most common view in regard to the relatively late admission of women to higher education in Germany is "the opinion, also voiced at the time, that Germany was 'backward' in terms of female education" (13). Mazón goes on to demonstrate that "[m]any scholars conflate this with the *Sonderweg* theory" (13).[58] The question of Germany being "backward" or different from other countries had already been addressed by Binder, Weber, and Morgenstern in the nineteenth century. This explanation alone, however, seems to be too simplistic to illuminate an issue that is quite complex. Mazón herself provides a convincing response to the question of why Germany opposed the entrance of women into universities for a much longer time than other European countries. She argues against the theories of Germany's "cultural or political backwardness" and claims that it was "the structure of German institutions" that caused woman's late admission (15). Specifically, Mazón focuses on the structure of the German research university and its close ties to the state. Unlike in many

57 Mazón points out that most female reformers although officially not associated with any potitical party "identified with the liberal end of the political spectrum" (6).

58 Mazón explains the Sonderweg theory as a theory "which refers to Germany's 'special path' to modernity, specifically to its failure to develop a viable modern parliamentary democracy before 1945" (13). See also her footnote regarding the definition (13; 232).

other European countries and in the United States, there were no private universities in Germany. Instead, the state financed all institutions of higher education (Mazón 6). This closed a venue of private individuals donating large sums of money for the purpose of women's admission or the possibility of establishing private universities for women (Mazón 6; 15). Drawing on the work by Jürgen Kocka, Mazón argues that in Germany "higher education, the state bureaucracy, and middle-class respectability were more closely intertwined than in other European countries" (6). The relation between the university and state was reciprocal. While the state financed the institutions of higher education, the university has been educating state employees for "the upper civil service" (Mazón 4). University-educated women could theoretically, as Mazón argues, demand access to "government jobs [...] and full participation in public life" (6). Because women were prohibited from joining political parties (until 1908) and did not have the right to vote (until 1918), providing women with higher education would, inevitably, lead to their claiming these civil rights as well (Mazón 2). In addition, as Mazón argues, the issue of higher education was closely tied to the question of middle-class identity, which was based, among other things, on an understanding of higher education as a "defining characteristic of its male members only" (Mazón 6).[59] What Mazón refers to as "the academic citizenship" included, according to her, much more than a physical presence at the university and acquisition of knowledge. It included, she argues, a particular life style, privileges, and obligations that were constitutive of middle-class masculinity. In addition to intellectual pursuit, heavy drinking, sexual relationships with prostitutes and women from lower social classes, debt, and dueling (Mazón 32; 35) constituted pillars of the student life, none of which were compatible with the nineteenth-century notion of middle-class femininity. As Mazón writes, "the image of the student was inseparable from, and indeed helped to create, the masculine identity of the educated middle class (46). The same image was a negation of everything that a middle-class woman was expected to be (Mazón 47-49).

59 At the same time, Mazón argues that Germany was not so "backward" in terms of higher education for women as many nineteenth-century intellectuals and contemporary scholars suggest. She writes: "Although many other European countries had admitted women by the 1870s, few universities could boast a significant number of female students, and in those that could, such as Paris or Zurich, most of the female students were foreigners" (14). In addition, she argues, several countries admitted women only to a few selected universities, but prohibited them from enrolling at others. At some universities (e.g. at Oxford) women could not "claim the degrees they had earned" (14). Seen from this perspective, Germany seems to have been more progressive: "In Germany, the discussion over women's higher education lasted longer, but the results were more uniform. Once a German state decided to admit women, all universities in that state had to do so. Thus, by 1909 all German universities were officially coeducational" (Mazón 14-15).

1.3 Major Arguments in the Debate about Women's Admission to Medical Schools

It is unquestionable that in the last decade of the nineteenth century higher education for women became a hotly debated topic. There were hardly any newspapers and magazines that did not engage in this discussion.[60] Similarly, a number of intellectuals, medical doctors, and scientists participated directly or indirectly in the public debate surrounding the admission of women to universities by writing specifically about female education, or more generally about restrictions placed on women by "nature." Two of the most (in)famous examples of discrediting women's cognitive ability were P.J. Möbius' *Über den physiologischen Schwachsinn des Weibes* and Otto Weininger's *Geschlecht und Charakter*. However, these widely read books are merely two of literally hundreds of other books, pamphlets, and articles written on this topic by both female and male authors.

In order to sample this wider debate, I will in this section give an overview of the major claims made by physicians, scientists, and members of the academic community pertaining to the admission of women to higher education. This will provide the ideological framework for my discussion of the politics of the female body in Germany and Austria at the end of the nineteenth century. The main focus of my analysis is a survey published in 1897 by Arthur Kirchhoff that contains essays and articles written by 122 university professors, doctors, teachers, and writers on "die Befähigung und Berechtigung des weiblichen Geschlechtes zum akademischen Studium" (Kirchhoff VII). Kirchhoff's survey illustrates the enormous public attention the possibility of higher education for women received and summarizes the various controversies the issue elicited. Although Kirchhoff himself supported the idea of women's higher education, he chose not to include or even mention in his publication any women who had written extensively on educational politics. By so doing, Kirchhoff sanctioned the exclusion of the female voice, even though his decision might have been well intended. Since the female voice did not have a substantial impact on any public decision-making until the issue of higher education had emerged, male support for the cause would have had a much stronger effect on the legislation.

The arguments presented by supporters and adversaries of women's admission to universities revolve around five major topics: (1) morality, (2) reproduction, (3) economics, (4) science and nature, and (5) tradition and social control.[61] Some arguments pertain to education in a university setting as such, while others

60 See also Mazón 97. For secondary literature regarding debates about education for women carried out in late-nineteenth-century press see Weiershausen 36.

61 Weiershausen summarizes main arguments in the debate by dividing them thematically as follows: (1) "Über die Befähigung der Frau zum wissenschaftlichen Studium und Berufe," (2) "Über den 'hohen, heiligen Beruf der Frau': Ehe und Familie," (3) "'Sittlichkeit und Frauenkeuschheit,'" and (4) "Die Akademikerin zwischen Krankheit, 'Entartung' und Unsittlichkeit" (41-59).

are targeted specifically at the medical field. Since they are directly or indirectly interrelated, I will provide a broad spectrum of opinions rather than referring only to those relevant to the medical field. I will show that the arguments of opponents of female education are concerned only on the surface with the good of women.[62] Anxiety over the imagined loss of female physical attractiveness resulting in the decrease of male sexual pleasure as well as the fear of economic losses emerge on the side of men as major sources of the hostility towards changes in the educational system.

1.3.1 Morality

The major claim pertaining to the standards of morality refers specifically to the medical profession. Opponents of female admission to medical schools employed arguments based on gender-specific norms of behavior and on the notion of prevailing moral standards.[63] The allocation of knowledge was gendered such that men were reared with access to different information than that available to women.[64] This pertains particularly to the knowledge about the anatomy and functions of the human body. While men were introduced to physiology in their adolescence, women were purposely kept ignorant in this regard. In the nineteenth century, the politics of education manifested itself especially in the realm of bourgeois sexuality. Middle-class men gained their pre-marital sexual experience in brothels or with women from lower social classes,[65] and middle-class women remained uninformed until the wedding night. Accordingly, medical knowledge was considered indecent and inappropriate for young middle-class women.[66] This constituted a big problem for medical schools, since, as Ziegeler puts it, women, if admitted, would be "in aller Öffentlichkeit mit Themen konfrontiert von denen sie *offiziell* nichts wissen durften" ("Zum Heile der Moral" 38). Hence, women's entrance into the public space of a medical school would constitute a transgression of knowledge boundaries (Ziegeler, "Zum Heile der Moral" 40).[67] Therefore, those

62 See also Weiershausen 48.

63 For a discussion of moral arguments see also Ziegeler, "Zum Heile der Moral" 36-42. See also Mazón 2.

64 Weiershausen also draws a similar conclusion: "Das Sittlichkeitsargument, das mit besonderem Nachdruck gegen das Medizinstudium von Frauen vorgebracht wurde, bestätigte schließlich die Annahme, daß es sich bei dem Wissen um Körper und Sexualität um einen geschlechtsspezifisch reglamentierten Bereich handelte" (58). See also Weiershausen 35.

65 Mazón points out that this was especially the case with university students (31-31). Hence, by entering universities women could be exposed to the lifestyle of male students and their sexual adventures. Here, an argument made by Griselda Pollock seems to be particularly relevant. She writes: "The guarded respectability of the lady could be soiled by mere visual contact for seeing what was bound up with knowing. The other world of encounter between bourgeois men and women of another class was a no-go area for bourgeois women" (78).

66 See also Weiershausen 52-53.

67 The question of epistemological boundaries will be addressed in Chapter Three.

in charge of academic curricula in many universities argued that admission of women would unavoidably lead to a transformation of existing university standards by adjusting lectures, books, and seminars to the level and form of knowledge socially acceptable for women.[68] This, in turn, would negatively influence the quality of male education.[69] It is clear from this line of argument that the assigned gender boundaries were perceived as a static entity and not as an object of social negotiation. The insistence on keeping women uninformed about their sexuality derived from male sexual fantasies about virgin women.[70] Tichy mentions that in the nineteenth century, the middle-class notion of virginity encompassed much more than a purely physical dimension ("Die geschlechtliche Un-Ordnung" 44-45). According to her, it also involved the lack of exposure to any sexual knowledge and unawareness of physical lovemaking which Rosa Mayreder called "[das] geistige Correlat der physischen Jungfräulichkeit" (qtd. in Tichy, "Die geschlechtliche Un-Ordnung" 44). In addition to chastity, the sexual ignorance of bourgeois women was considered to be very appealing to the male tastes of the time (Tichy, "Die geschlechtliche Un-Ordnung" 44-45). Thus, male sexual pleasure seems to have been one driving force behind the insistence on keeping women sexually uninformed and, consequently, a factor in the resistance to admission of women to medical schools.[71]

In addition to excluding women from medical schools, arguments employing the notion of prevailing moral standards perpetuated female physical and mental virginity and secured male dominance in spheres other than the sexual as well. One of the participants in Kirchhoff's survey, Professor Georg Lewin, makes this connection explicit:

> *Die echte Weiblichkeit, die uns nicht allein 'hinanzieht,' sondern vor allem zur Liebe i.e. zur Heirat bewegt, wird, wenn sie nicht durch jenes anstrengende konkrete Studium ganz zu Grunde geht, doch beschädigt. Dies ist vor allem beim Studium der Medizin der Fall.*

---

68 Mazón also points out that some professors "saw women as a danger to the university's standards" (102).

69 See also Heindl, "Zur Entwicklung des Frauenstudiums" 19.

70 Tichy also points out that "eine Bedrohung von Phantasien" ("Die geschlechtliche Un-Ordnung" 29) seemed to be a motivating factor behind the resistance to medical education of women. She further writes: "Was mit dem Anspruch der Frauen auf die Wissenschaft grundsätzlich zur Debatte stand, waren die Denk- und Wahrnehmungsmuster, auf denen die Weiblichkeitsmythen der bürgerlichen Kultur jener Zeit beruhten, in ihrer Totalität" ("Die geschlechtliche Un-Ordnung" 29-30).

71 Tichy writes: "Erst in Anbetrachten des männlichen Monopols auf das Wissen über den eigenen und den weiblichen Körper werden die auffallend starken Ressentiments nachvollziehbar, die sich gegen das Medizinstudium von Frauen richten und in Wittels' Kommentar zum 'Eindringen des Weibes ins Laboratorium' und bösartig-kastrierenden 'Kathederweib' beredten Ausdruck finden" ("Die geschlechtliche Un-Ordnung" 45). I will elaborate on her discussion of Wittels' article and develop this argument in Chapter Three.

Eine Frau, die über die Anatomie der Geschlechtsteile nicht allein des Weibes, sondern auch des Mannes orientiert ist und über das Mysterium des Geschlechtsaktes ohne Erröten sprechen kann, wird den Mann, wenn nicht immer abstoßen, so doch immer kalt lassen. (Kirchhoff 73)

The link between the acquisition of knowledge by women and the loss of their physical attractiveness[72] made by opponents of female education will be explored later. At this point, however, I want to emphasize the importance of the female body and its status as a sexual object in the debate.

The second moral argument employed in the campaign against the admission of women to universities saw in coeducation a threat to students' moral conduct. According to the authorities of the university in Vienna, men and women sharing the same classrooms while attending lectures and seminars would pose "große Gefahren für den wissenschaftlichen und sittlichen Ernst beider [Geschlechter]" (*Gutachten des Akademischen Senats der Universität Wien/1873* qtd. in Heindl, "Zur Entwicklung des Frauenstudiums" 19). Similarly, Victor Birch-Hirschfeld argued in Kirchhoff's survey:

Gewisse Fachstudien, namentlich in Form der Praktika, können gar nicht in unbefangener Weise vor einem gemischten Publikum behandelt werden. Dagegen würde sich auch das Zartgefühl gerade des besten Teils unserer deutschen Studenten auflehnen. Sie sind nun einmal in der Auffassung edler Weiblichkeit aufgewachsen, die es schwer macht, in der Medizinstudentin ein gewissermaßen neutrales Individuum mit den äußeren Attributen des Weiblichen zu ertragen. (Kirchhoff 64)

As suggested by this passage, the notion of "edle Weiblichkeit" is based on woman's ignorance regarding sexuality and her lack of knowledge regarding functions of the human body. Furthermore, Birch-Hirschfeld points out the distinction between a real woman and an individual with external feminine features. This distinction is very important for the debate about admission of women to medical schools. Women aspiring to higher education were believed to be less feminine than other women because the desire for knowledge itself was supposed to be foreign to female nature.[73] Hence, even if women were able to maintain physical feminine characteristics while studying at a university, which presumably all

---

72 Tichy refers to this phenomenon as "[d]er phantasierte Antagonismus zwischen Weiblichkeit und akademischer Ausbildung" ("Die geschlechtliche Un-Ordnung" 39). See also Tichy, "Die geschlechtliche Un-Ordnung" 38.

73 This connection has been emphasized by many scholars writing on the subject. See, for example, Weiershausen's discussion of "Konfrontation von 'Weiblichkeit' und Wissenschaft" (9) throughout her book.

women did, they were not seen as real women but rather as "mental hermaphrodites."[74] At the same time, many professors admitted that their own insecurity would not allow them to conduct lectures and seminars in front of a coeducational audience.[75]

The supporters of female medical education employed different but related moral arguments. They emphasized feminine feelings of shame in the case of medical examination by a male doctor.[76] This argument gained even more importance in the Austro-Hungarian Empire, especially in Bosnia and Herzegovina with their Moslem population.[77] The proponents drew public attention to the traumatic experience an examination by a male doctor would cause in girls and young women.[78] In this regard, the legislative authorities showed a willingness to consider employment of female doctors in schools for girls (Ziegeler, "Zum Heile der Moral" 33).[79] Another area potentially opened to female doctors by such concern for morality was a role as *Sittenpolizei* responsible for the examination and arrest of women suspected of prostitution (Ziegeler, *Weibliche Ärzte* 37).[80] Although I will discuss the specific women's positions regarding these arguments in detail later, I would like to quote Rosa Mayreder, an outspoken supporter of female education, on the issue of morality because her statement summarizes very accurately the opposing opinions. She pointed out logical fallacies in the reasoning of the conservative side; a lack of knowledge of the human body, suppression of sexuality, and feelings of shame that are supposed to constitute true femininity do not go hand in hand with medical examination of women by male doctors:

> Da wird uns beständig vorgeflötet, dass das Schamgefühl die edelste Zierde eines edlen Weibes sei usw; wenn es sich aber darum handelt, praktische Konsequenzen zu ziehen, dann schweigen diese Flöten. Denn ohne Zweifel gehört die Behandlung durch einen männlichen Arzt in vielen Krankheitsfällen zu den schmerzlichsten Beleidigungen des weiblichen Schamgefühls. [...] [M]an konnte in den letzten [Debatten] sehr häufig hören, dass die meisten Frauen sich ganz gerne durch einen männlichen Arzt behandeln lassen. Also

---

74 Thorson uses the term "the spiritual hermaphrodite" (69). Robert Michels uses the term "geistige Hermaphroditen" in 1902 (qtd. in Tichy, "Die geschlechtliche Un-Ordnung" 35).

75 Burchardt 14, 16-17; Bandhauer-Schöffmann 66-67; see also Mazón 1.

76 For a more detailed discussion of such arguments among the members of AÖF see Bandhauer-Schöffmann 53-55; 63. See also Ziegeler, "Zum Heile der Moral" 36-38; Hoesch 46; Ziegeler, *Weibliche Ärzte* 111-30; Glaser, "Die erste Studentinnengeneration" 311; Weiershausen 52; Schmersahl 303.

77 Bandhauer-Schöffmann 53; Ziegeler, "Zum Heile der Moral" 33.

78 See also Ziegeler "Zum Heile der Moral" 34.

79 For a detailed discussion of the issue of school physicians for girls see Ziegeler, *Weibliche Ärzte* 27-32.

80 For a detailed discussion of the employment of female physicians by the *Sittenpolizei* see Ziegeler, *Weibliche Ärzte* 37-44.

> entweder ist der hohe Grad weiblicher Schamhaftigkeit nur eine Legende, oder man spricht nur davon, wenn es einem gerade in den Kram paßt. (qtd. in Bandhauer-Schöffmann 59-60)

Mayreder points out that the opponents of female medical education used their moral arguments strategically to legitimate male dominance in society, in general, and in the medical field, in particular. Many male physicians supported Mayreder's statement, admitting that the examination of women by male doctors could indeed constitute a distressing experience for the patient. They also emphasized that the anxiety over such an examination could cause women not to consult a doctor in case of an illness.[81] However, not all physicians were ready to accept this argument, because it would have had far-reaching consequences for the entire medical profession, the most important being the opening of medical schools to women. They appealed to male authority by assuming that the male doctor will always be more competent than the female one. [82]

1.3.2 Reproduction

The set of claims in Kirchhoff's survey pertaining to reproduction focuses on the notion of motherhood. At the same time, the female reproductive function emerges in the debates almost as a justification for the existence of women. Men, on the contrary, did not need any justification, since the raison d'être of their existence was believed to be self-explanatory. These arguments were concerned with women's access to higher education in general and were, with one exception, not restricted to medical schools. The question of motherhood was discussed not only on a personal level, but even more importantly on a national level, by equating the issue to the fate of the nation. The ability or willingness of women to have children became a question of the reproductive capacity of the nation. Consequently, women who willingly jeopardized their ability to give birth were judged in terms of their patriotism. Since the participation of women in higher education was believed to endanger their reproductive functions, the opponents of women's admission to medical schools elevated the issue to the question of national interests. According to many physicians and academics, women's higher education and childbearing functions were mutually exclusive, and since reproduction was considered to be the one and only social role women had to fulfill, the demand for higher education emerged in this light as merely an unreasonable whim. The nationalistic rhetoric is evident in a statement by Isidor Rosenthal, who perceived the establishment of high schools for girls as "ein nationales Unglück" (Kirchhoff 54). According to this line of argument, admission of women to the universities would only distract them from their true service to the family and to the nation.

---

81 See, for example, the statement made by Robert Olshausen (Kirchhoff 121).

82 See, for example, the statement made by Adolf Kehrer (Kirchhoff 114).

Following this logic, the proponents of female education also tried to use family and nation to provide reasons and justifications for opening high schools for women. Therefore, arguments supporting female education evolved around the advantages that not only men but also the whole nation would gain from women's admission to universities. Ottomar Rosenbach, for example, argued that an educated woman would be a better wife and mother,[83] and secondly, such a woman would be more likely to give birth to and rear great men:[84]

> Wir haben [...] durchaus kein Recht die Befähigung der Frauen unseres Landes zu unterschätzen, [...] *da die geistige Befähigung vieler hervorragenden Männer eine Gabe der Mütter zu sein scheint, und da wohl bei den besten Söhnen der Nation nachweislich die Mutter hervorragend erzieherisch gewirkt hat.* Diese Funktion wird sie im Vollbesitze des Wissens ihrer Zeit noch besser erfüllen als bisher, und die geistigen Fähigkeiten und Leistungen der Nachkommen werden also nach dem *Entwicklungsgesetze* noch gesteigert werden. (Kirchhoff 80)

According to this argument, women's education was not an aim in itself, but rather it constituted only a means to the ultimate goal—the better qualifications and achievements of male citizens. In a related argument and referring specifically to medical education, supporters emphasized the necessity of educating female gynecologists for the good of the nation. They pointed out that many women died or suffered severe impairments because they refused to go to a male doctor. Consequently, by rejecting female doctors, Germany and Austria jeopardized the reproductive health of the nation.

1.3.3 Economics

Arguments pertaining to the economy in Kirchhoff's collection emphasize difficulties in obtaining a job in the medical profession at the end of the nineteenth century.[85] The opponents of female education pointed out that there were already

83 See also Weiershausen 51-52. In addition, Weiershausen points out that "[d]ie Differenzierung zwischen einem Studium zu reinen Bildungszwecken und einem, das auf eine spätere Berufsausübung abzielt, war ein wichtiger Aspekt in der Debatte über das Frauenstudium" (51). Referring to an argument made by Edith Glaser and Ulrich Hermann, Weiershausen demonstrates that the admission of women to higher education for the sake of gaining general knowledge did not generate as much controversy as the admission for the sake of professional development (51). Mazón maintains that also "[o]pponents of female students argued that women's education should aim to produce competent wives and mothers but not extend beyond this" (5).

84 See also the argument made by Leo Reinisch (qtd. in Heindl, "Zur Entwicklung des Frauenstudiums in Österreich" 21).

85 See also Tichy, "Die geschlechtliche Un-Ordnung" 27-29; Ziegeler, *Weibliche Ärzte* 25-26.

too many physicians and an additional number of female medical students would certainly not improve the situation.[86] Victor Birch-Hirschfeld, a participant in Kirchhoff's survey, combined the argument of a lack of medical jobs with that of female inferiority:

> Da nun bereits seit Jahren [...] eine über das wirtschaftliche Bedürfnis hinausgehende Produktion von Ärzten stattgefunden hat, die es [...] schwerer macht, eine ausreichende Lebensstellung zu gewinnen, so wäre es unverantwortlich, wenn man jetzt durch Zulassung weiblicher Ärzte die Konkurrenz durch [...] doch im allgemeinen minderwertige Mitbewerber steigern wollte. *Der Vorteil, daß auf diese Weise vielleicht einige Tausende unbeschäftigter weiblicher Arbeitskräfte aus den gebildeten Ständen unterzubringen wären, würde mehr als aufgewogen durch die wirtschaftliche Schädigung, die durch derartige "billige" Mitbewerber den Ärzten und den von letzteren abhängigen Familiengliedern zugefügt würde.* (Kirchhoff 63)

As clearly illustrated by Birch-Hirschfeld, male job security had priority over the establishment of a means of existence for single bourgeois women, who in most cases were considered a financial burden for their relatives and needed a source of income to be able to live. Since unmarried women did not fulfill the reproductive function, they also did not have much social value. The second part of Birch-Hirschfeld's argument focused on women as generally inferior candidates on the job market and implied a lack of any social benefits from admitting women to medical schools.

The economic arguments employed by supporters of female education centered inevitably on the necessity of providing sources of income for single middle-class women and pointed out, utilizing a great deal of pathos, the inhumanity of the decision to deny a basis of existence to these women.[87] However, the

86 Ziegler argues that there was no real threat of the labor market overflowing with unemployed medical doctors. Instead, she claims, the fears of potential unemployment expressed by male physicians were completely irrational, based on a generally perceived threat of social changes caused by the admission of women to universities (*Weibliche Ärzte* 25). Tichy maintains that "eine Bedrohung von Phantasien" was a much more important motivation than "die männliche Realangst vor einer möglichen Konkurenz auf dem Arbeitsmarkt" ("Die geschlechtliche Un-Ordnung" 29). Weiershausen claims that "die Furcht vor einer Ärzteschwemme" was prevalent at the end of the nineteenth century. However, she also shows by referring to Claudia Huerkamp's argument that this fear was not grounded in social reality (39). See also Schmersahl 303-304. Mazón stresses the "fear of professional competition with women" (103). See also Mazón 5; 93-94.

87 See also Glaser, "Die erste Studentinnengeneration" 313; and the argument made by Leo Reinisch and Marianne Hainisch (qtd. in Heindl, "Zur Entwicklung des Frauenstudiums in Österreich" 21-23).

demand to open universities to women was focused not solely on unmarried women, but also emphasized the necessity of financial independence for all women. Albert Moll, among others, tied this argument in with the critique of the institution of bourgeois marriage. He argued that only women from well-off families had a chance to get married. In marriage, they were financially completely dependent on their husbands and did not have any autonomy. The pressure to marry for financial reasons puts this kind of marriage in the same category as prostitution (Kirchhoff 138).

1.3.4 Science and Nature

The main arguments against female education in Kirchhoff's survey emphasized women's intellectual inferiority, which supposedly made intellectual work impossible.[88] Along the same lines, it was argued that intellectual work was against female nature. The physical weakness of the female body supposedly posed an obstacle especially with regard to the medical profession. Thus the majority of doctors and scientists defined women as physically and intellectually incapable of studying medicine.[89]

The pamphlets and articles against female education usually presented two hypothetical situations: women who are not able to overcome their nature expose themselves to ridicule in their pursuit of higher education, or if they persist, they become students but lose their feminine aspect and acquire masculine characteristics. According to this logic, two female student types appeared in the public discourse and were ridiculed.[90] Margit Brunner and Eva Brinkschulte, who investigated the question of women's education in late nineteenth and early twentieth century, presented examples of both types of caricatures in their publications.

One of these caricatures depicts a female medical student during an examination standing in front of a half-naked female patient. Both women are surrounded by physicians and medical students. The caption lampoons the situation: "Kandidatin, sagen Sie mir, was fällt Ihnen an der Patientin auf?" – "Daß der Mensch einen seidenen Unterrock anhat" (Brinkschulte, *Weibliche Ärzte* 23). This exchange obviously presents a stereotype about women who were generally believed to think only about superficial things such as clothing and jewelry. Brunner reprints another caricature of a woman showing her breasts publicly. The caption reads: "Die ehemalige Studentin im Berufsalltag" (85). Both caricatures refer to

---

88 Tichy writes: "Zwangsläufig muß die bürgerliche Weiblichkeitskonzeption, die die körperliche Unfähigkeit der Frau zur Intellektualität als Regel aufgestellt hat, weibliche Intellektuelle als Ausnahmen, die die Regel bestätigen, kategorisieren" ("Die geschlechtliche Un-Ordnung" 35).

89 See also Tichy, "Die geschlechtliche Un-Ordnung" 29-78; Rohner 66-67; Weiershausen 41-45.

90 The discussion of the female student and her representation will be developed in Chapter Three.

the first hypothetical situation in which women are presented as being unable to overcome either their "natural feminine traits" such as lack of cognition and superficiality, or their strong sensual and sexual nature.

Other caricatures depict female students as ugly women with glasses and thinning hair (reprinted in Brunner 83-84) who obviously have lost their feminine body features and consequently their "decorative" value.[91] These kinds of images focus on the aesthetic aspect of the female body and clearly evoke a discourse about value: these women have lost their value on the marriage market. Their entry into the public space of a university becomes discursively inscribed into the surface of their bodies. In these caricatures, the surface of the female body provides a visible manifestation of the developed intellect as an abnormal feature.

The obsession of male writers with the female body as the embodiment of man's visual and sexual pleasure is manifested in the notion that knowledge is capable of physically deforming female bodies. Many physicians, for instance, believed that the learning process influenced female health in a negative way.[92] Karl von Bardeleben argued that numerous hours spent sitting and learning would potentially create in women "*schädliche Einwirkungen auf die Wirbelsäule und auf den Brustkorb, auch das Becken, ferner auf die Zirkulationsorgane* und vor allem auf *die Unterleibsorgane*" (Kirchhoff 33).

In addition, many opponents of education for women brought up the alleged lack of cognitive abilities in females. Bardeleben voiced a popular belief that "die Begabung des Weibes für das Studium [...] im Durchschnitt eine *geringere* ist, als die der Männer" (Kirchhoff 34). Gustav Fritsch argued in a similar way: "Mit dieser zarteren Natur [der Frau] hängt wohl auch die häufig recht mangelhaft entwickelte Gabe des Gedächtnisses zusammen" (Kirchhoff 46). He agreed that there are some women who perform relatively well as students; however, they are only exceptions and not the rule (Kirchhoff 45). Many, like Birch-Hirschfeld, argued that so-called feminine characteristics like tenderness, feeling, and compassion are important for a physician. However, these characteristics are not sufficient for entrance into the medical profession (Kirchhoff 62-63). This debate polarizes gender characteristics of compassion and feelings in the feminine realm, and self-control, clarity of thought, independence, and determination in the masculine realm. In this configuration, according to Birch-Hirschfeld, only the male is capable of evoking a patient's trust:

> Darf man den weiblichen Beruf zur Krankenpflege aus den mütterlichen Eigenschaften des Weibes herleiten, so beruht die ärztliche Tüchtigkeit – namentlich soweit sie in dem Einfluß der Autorität des Arztes wurzelt, auf männlicher, ja man kann sagen 'väterlicher' Begabung. (Kirchhoff 63)

---

91 While describing a different image, Brunner refers to "Frau als schmückendes Element" (84).

92 See also Burchardt 10-11; Schmersahl 305; 312-313.

Birch-Hirschfeld takes recourse to stereotypical gender roles in the family and implies that this polarization encompasses not only the private, but also the public sphere. Since the father figure is usually associated with respect and decision-making, and the mother figure with love and compassion, Birch-Hirschfeld argues that the patient seeks treatment of illnesses from a male doctor, but expects merely compassion from a female one. This argument clearly shows that trust does not have much to do with education but with the deeply rooted perception of gender roles.

The supporters of female education, such as Albert Eulenburg, argued against this conviction, but they also confirmed, although less aggressively, the notion of gender difference:

> Wenn man also mit einer gewissen Berechtigung aussprechen kann, daß im allgemeinen beim Manne Verstand und logisches Denken, beim Weibe Gefühl und sinnliches Empfinden überwiegen, so ist damit noch keineswegs gesagt, daß gerade letztere Eigenschaften die Frauen für wissenschaftliches Studium, zumal auf medizinischem Gebiete, als minder befähigt erscheinen ließen. (Kirchhoff 130)

Others pointed out that individual differences play a much more substantial role than gender differences. Julius Bernstein addressed the issue of the assumed inferior physical construction of women in addition to cognitive or emotional faculties. He denied the validity of this premise by pointing to the hardships of various kinds of work that women in the lower classes have to undertake:

> Viele Männer würden den Anstrengungen, denen eine Waschfrau, viele Ärzte den Strapazen, denen eine Hebamme ausgesetzt ist, nicht gewachsen sein. Und was die geistigen Fähigkeiten anbetrifft, so verhält es sich mit diesen entschieden ebenso. Wollten wir aus solchen Gründen die Ergreifung des Berufes verbieten, so müßten wir auch einer großen Zahl von Männern in dieser Beziehung Beschränkungen auferlegen. *Ob das Weib zu irgend einem Berufe geeignet ist, läßt sich m. E. a priori nicht entscheiden; hierüber kann nur die Erfahrung Auskunft geben*, und diese wird lehren, ob das Weib dem Manne im Kampfe ums Dasein gewachsen ist. (Kirchhoff 42)

Indeed, the main argument employed by the supporters of female medical education utilized the "female nature theory" to show that women are better caregivers than men. Robert Olshausen emphasized: "die zartere Hand der Frau, [...] ihr zarteres Gemüt und Gefühl" (Kirchhoff 121). However, according to Olshausen, these qualities were believed to be of special importance only "im Gebiet der Frauen- und Kinderheilkunde" (Kirchhoff 121). Thus, even the arguments utilized by supporters of female medical education were rooted in gender stereotypes. It was still unthinkable that female doctors might treat male patients.[93] Because the relationship between the doctor and the patient was also a power relation, in which the doctor was in total control of the patient's passive body, the reversal of traditional gender roles (passive female and active male) that would take place in such a situation was unacceptable to the majority.

1.3.5 Tradition and Social Control

As I have already pointed out, Russian women constituted the majority of female medical students in Zurich in the 1860s and early 1870s. A contemporary historian Hanny Rohner cites two main reasons for their prevalence. Although there had been high schools for girls in Russia since the 1850s, it was not until the 1870s that any universities were open to women. In addition, many young people influenced by Marx's revolutionary ideas wanted to spread these, and the study of medicine in Zurich provided a good excuse for going abroad.[94] Revolutionary activities were strictly prohibited in Russia, as censorship made it very difficult to propagate new ideas, and the repressive state crushed any political clubs. In this situation, it was easier to develop revolutionary activities abroad directed against the Russian system. According to Rohner "im Sommer 1873 [befanden sich] unter 114 Studentinnen 100 Russinnen, welche sich aber nur zum kleinen Teil ernsthaften Studien widmeten" (15). Although the Russian government prohibited women from studying abroad in 1873 and demanded that all female students return to Russia immediately, the impression left by them remained and influenced the reputation of all female students.[95] This situation provided new arguments against the admission of women to the universities in Europe that Bertha von Suttner summarized as follows: "[S]o entstand in der Vorstellung der Menge eine Vermischung der Begriffe Nihilismus und weibliches Studententum: eine Ideenverbindung, die umso natürlicher war, als beides auf Befreiungsprinzipien beruhte" (qtd. in Heindl, "Die russischen Studentinnen" 131). The demands to reevaluate gender roles and to implement necessary changes in the educational system evoked, as confirmed by Suttner, an association of female students with nihilism, socialism, and anarchism. Accordingly, most of the arguments employed against the admission of women to universities were fueled by the desire to preserve the existing social order. Franz Riegel maintained that "[d]er Frauen

---

93 Ziegeler, *Weibliche Ärzte* 30-31; Ziegeler, "Zum Heile der Moral" 38; Hoesch 45. See also Mazón 59; 107.

94 Rohner 15; Heindl, "Die russischen Studentinnen" 131-132.

95 Rohner 16; Heindl, "Zur Entwicklung des Frauenstudiums" 19; Heindl, "Die russischen Studentinnen" 131; Burchardt 21. See also Mazón 60-62; 94; Weiershausen 55-57. Weiershausen demonstrates that some opponents of medical education for women speculated that women wanted to pursue the study of medicine in order to learn how to perform abortions. These accusations, as Weiershausen argues, were false (56-57).

höchstes Ziel muß der häusliche Herd, das Familienheim bleiben, soll anders die Weltordnung nicht verschoben werden" (Kirchhoff 77). Karl Lemayer based his argument against admitting women to universities on his belief that "ein gutes Geschick" had excluded women from most professions. He argued that the exclusion of women from the universities would prove the best possible good for society:

> [S]o lange die Gesellschaft, was ein gutes Geschick verhüten möge, die Frauen nicht als Priester, Richter, Advokaten, Ärzte, Lehrer, Feldherrn, Krieger aufzunehmen das Bedürfnis hat, das heißt, so lange der Schwerpunkt der Leitung der sozialen Ordnung noch in dem männlichen Geschlecht ruht, liegt auch keine Nötigung vor, den Frauen an der Universität ein Terrain einzuräumen, welches in den weiteren Folgen unmöglich zu begrenzen wäre. (qtd. in Heindl, "Zur Entwicklung des Frauenstudiums in Österreich" 19-20)

According to Lemayer, the status quo guaranteed the continuation of the best possible social order. Any changes, it is clearly implied, were going to lead to chaos and disaster. Riegel's and Lemayer's remarks, when placed in the appropriate sociohistorical context, shed more light on the deep roots of the resistance to opening university gates for women. The social order to which both Riegel and Lemayer referred was German bourgeois society of the eighteenth and nineteenth centuries. The strict differentiation between male (state) and female (family) domains within the middle-class was, as Ute Frevert demonstrated, one of the building blocks of the German bourgeois society.[96] Frevert argued that the division of society in "weibliche [...] und männliche [...] Menschen" (22) was deeply rooted in German political and social thought of the eighteenth and nineteenth centuries as the most influential German thinkers and theorists of civil society, such as Kant, Fichte, Schlegel, and Hegel had excluded women in their theoretical writings from any participation in the matters of the state. It was more than obvious for these thinkers that women were "grundsätzlich und unveränderlich außerhalb des politisch-rechtlichen Zusammenhangs bürgerlicher Gesellschaften" (Frevert 22). As a result, as Frevert puts it,

> Von Kant bis Hegel – und weit darüber hinaus – zog sich somit die Vorstellung von zwei faktisch und idealisch getrennten Wirkungsbereichen der Geschlechter durch die theoretischen Entwürfe bürgerlicher Gesellschaft. [...] Alle Glorifikationen und Idyllisierungen der Weiblichkeit [...] änderten nichts an dem Grundsatz funktionaler

96 Ute Frevert. "Bürgerliche Meisterdenker und das Geschlechterverhältnis. Konzepte, Erfahrungen, Visionen and der Wende vom 18. zum 19. Jahrhundert." *Bürgerinnen und Bürger. Gerschlechterverhältnisse im 19. Jahrhundert.* Ed. Ute Frevert. Göttingen: Vandenhoeck u. Ruprecht, 1988. 17-48.

> Differenzierung der "Menschheit" in zwei Geschlechter, der als elementares Ordnungsprinzip bürgerlicher Gesellschaft übernommen wurde. (30-31)

Since political and social writings by philosophers such as Kant, Fichte, Schlegel, and Hegel constituted "einen Kanon bürgerlicher Selbstverständigung, mit dem sich Generationen von Bildungsbürgern kritisch und affirmativ auseinandersetzten" (Frevert 19), it was the very core of "bürgerlicher Selbstverständigung" that was at stake in the debate about women's admission to higher education. Several other scholars emphasized the connection between the ideology of the bourgeois society and the resistance to women's demands. Schmersahl, for example, argued that the nineteenth-century medicine only legitimized the social order of German bourgeois society (Schmersahl 1) and Mazón emphasized throughout her work "the close relationship between the university, the state, and [...] society as a whole" (105).[97]

1.4 Female Responses to Kirchhoff's Survey

Although Kirchhoff chose not to include any women in his survey, it elicited female responses. Helene Lange and Käthe Schirmacher reacted critically in the feminist press. Both wrote reviews of the survey and used them as a vehicle to represent the progressive female voice not only in matters of higher education as such, but also in regard to gender politics in Germany. They showed that a social construct of gender characteristics, and not a woman's alleged lack of intellectual abilities, hindered women in their pursuit of an academic education. In addition, they demanded that the female voice should play the decisive role in the debate and decision-making regarding women's higher education. Simultaneously, they critically evaluated the competence and qualifications of the participants in Kirchhoff's survey to make seemingly profound statements about female education.

As indicated by the title of Kirchhoff's survey, *Die akademische Frau. Gutachten hervorragender Universitätsprofessoren, Frauenlehrer und Schriftsteller über die Befähigung der Frau zum Studium und Berufe*, his intention was to collect and publish experts' opinions. Lange and Schirmacher, however, pointed out that most of the participants in Kirchhoff's survey had never taught or even interacted with female students and their opinions were therefore merely theoretical speculations. Lange writes:

> [D]ie meisten Urteile des vorliegenden Buches sind [...] nicht auf Erfahrung, Induktion, Experiment gegründet, sondern auf Hypothese, Deduktion, Theorie oder auf gar nichts. Neben streng logisch aus ersten Gründen hergeleiteten Deduktionen finden wir darunter auch

97 See also Weiershausen 33; 39-40.

> jene öden, unbewiesenen Allgemeinheiten, die den Mangel eigener Gedanken bemänteln. Die positive Bedeutung des Buches für das Frauenstudium ist damit ungefähr umschrieben. ("Die akademische Frau" 194)

As stated in this passage, assumptions, theories, and subjective personal opinions replaced facts, evidence, and practical experience. According to Lange, there is no point in arguing and speculating theoretically whether women are capable of studying in an academic environment and whether such activity would affect them in a negative way. Such speculations do not prove female skills and ability to work intellectually. They are merely intellectual games showing the deduction and logical thinking skills of the survey participants. They do not establish the basis either for admitting women to universities or for excluding them from higher education. On the contrary, they show varying degrees of openness to progressive ideas and social changes among German academics (Lange, "Die akademische Frau" 194). In addition, Lange shows that teachers and professors who had taught women and therefore had practical knowledge in these matters generally support female higher education based on their positive experiences. They do not perceive women as inferior candidates for higher education and they do not see any valid reason for excluding them from universities. Lange refers to countries that had already admitted women to universities to show that an informed decision can be based only on knowledge derived from practical experience. According to Lange, the New Hospital for Women in London was a good example of an institution established and directed by women, in which female physicians conducted difficult surgeries every day. In addition, there were many colleges not only in Great Britain but also in other European countries in which women proved to be successful as professors and as students. In Germany, scientists, writers, and teachers debated the issue theoretically instead of allowing women to enter universities in order to find out whether they would actually be successful or not (Lange, "Die akademische Frau" 194). Lange does not see any point in debating higher education for women in Germany, since only empirical evidence can provide relevant answers to the question.

Although the vast majority of the surveyed professors and writers support, at least partially, higher education for women, Lange questions the relevance of Kirchhoff's survey in general, because it does not contribute to a solution of the problem. Further, she demonstrates that adversaries of female education could not uphold their theories when confronted with concrete examples. Three main arguments used against female education, particularly in the medical field, (the physiology of the female body, its delicate build, and woman's function as wife and mother) have been proven false through experience and the demonstrated abilities of many women around the world, according to Lange. Schirmacher too, indicates the pointlessness of Kirchhoff's survey, referring to a lack of practical experience in Germany and to the wide range of opinions regarding this issue:

> So durchlaufen wir denn die Reihe aller nur möglichen Urteile: die Frau ist weniger zum Studium befähigt, als der Mann; sie ist ebenso befähigt; sie ist für gewisse Fächer besser befähigt. Angesichts dieser fortwährenden Widersprüche muß man diejenigen eigentlich für die Weisesten halten, die da sagen: Wir haben heute noch gar kein Urteil über die Befähigung der Frau zum akademischen Studium und müssen deshalb in dieser Hinsicht erst Erfahrungen sammeln, d.h. die Frauen studieren lassen. ("Die akademische Frau" 4)

Both Lange and Schirmacher emphasize the inconsistency of arguments and the lack of uniformity among German academics who wrote "die unvereinbarsten Dinge" (Lange, "Die akademische Frau" 194) about a woman's ability to pursue intellectual work. This inconsistency of opinions and arguments derives mainly from varying degrees of practical experience (or lack thereof) on the side of German academics, they argue; only professors who never interacted with female students are the most fervent opponents of higher education for women.

In addition to the experience factor, Lange indicated that members of certain academic disciplines were more inclined than others to oppose female education. According to Lange, professors of medicine and philology were the most zealous adversaries. The explanation seems obvious to her: medical doctors and philology professors felt threatened because their fields have had the biggest appeal to women. Schirmacher also emphasizes the competition factor:

> Die Hauptangriffe gehen überhaupt nicht gegen die Frau als Prediger, Richter und Professor, sondern gegen die Frau als Arzt. – Das liegt zum Teil wohl daran, daß die Frau erstere Berufe noch nicht ernstlich zu bedrohen scheint, im ärztlichen Beruf aber bereits drinsteht und Konkurrent ist. ("Die akademische Frau" 16)

Lange stresses that two of the three gynecologists participating in Kirchhoff's survey proved to be the most fanatical opponents. Yet this particular branch of medicine demonstrated the greatest demand for female physicians (Lange, "Die akademische Frau" 197).

Medicine as a potential professional field for women elicited the most responses in Kirchhoff's survey. And again, it revealed the lack of concurrence among participants. Schirmacher concludes that faced with such major discrepancies in arguments and inconsistencies among male "experts," the women's voice should be decisive in the final decision regarding female medical education in Germany. She indicates that Kirchhoff based his survey on two false premises: he assumed that university professors are the best experts regarding female education although most of them did not have any experience with female students, and he chose not to consider the opinion of women, who were directly affected by this debate. Hence, Schirmacher points out, women are being denied autonomy in decision-making:

> [M]an muß da eben die Nächstbeteiligten zu Rate ziehen und Versuche machen lassen. Die Nächstbeteiligten aber sind die Frauen, und heute steht es bereits fest, sowohl daß Frauen Arzt sein können, wie daß Frauen weibliche Ärzte haben wollen. Gewiß, nicht alle Frauen können Arzt sein, nicht alle Frauen wünschen sich von weiblichen Ärzten behandeln zu lassen; aber eine bestimmte Anzahl kann es und will es, und dieser Anzahl soll es überlassen bleiben, Angebot und Nachfrage, wie sie will, zu regeln. ("Die akademische Frau" 17)

Both the experience with medical education for women in other countries and the necessity for university access articulated by German women should be sufficient to silence the opponents and to reach a consensus in the debate.

Moreover, Schirmacher hints at the tendency of opponents of female education to use abstract concepts instead of specific examples in the debate. Their arguments refer very often to the abstract idea of "woman" and hence to all women in general. The opponents do not take women as individual beings into consideration, but regard them as part of a "species-woman." She emphasizes that women are individuals with different skills, abilities, and preferences and cannot be treated as a uniform mass. While the adversaries of female education seem to refer to men and women as two more or less distinct yet uniform groups of people, the supporters look at individuals instead. The former perceive each woman as representative of all women; the latter see a woman as an individual competing with another individual, male or female. In other words, a concrete female individual is juxtaposed with woman as an abstract concept. Schirmacher dismisses the theories that proclaim inherent differences between male and female mental faculties and the theories that define all women as intellectually inferior. She states: "[D]erselbe Mangel findet sich ebenso bei Männern, und bei den betreffenden Individuen beider Geschlechter kann er durch Erziehung gehoben werden" (Schirmacher, "Die akademische Frau" 3).

Both Schirmacher and Lange make it very clear that the reason for closing the university gates on women is not their alleged lack of intellectual abilities but rather a socially constructed image of gender characteristics. Some German women already fulfill all academic requirements, but university authorities and professors still discriminate against them on the basis of their gender. Although almost all participants in Kirchhoff's survey agree that an *Abitur* should qualify women for admission to a university, Schirmacher asks why, in this case, all eight Prussian women who had passed the *Abitur* were not admitted to a single university ("Die akademische Frau" 15). To demonstrate gendered social consciousness, she quotes Berthold Delbrück, a professor of philology, who admitted that if one of his female Sanskrit students had been a man, he would have recommended her for a *Habilitation* at the university. This admission shows that despite demonstrated aptitude and excellent educational results, women were unable to pursue their academic interests due to the general views about gender. It is social perception of gender and not lack of intellectual abilities that hindered women in their pursuit.

Kirchhoff's decision not to include any women in his survey might actually have been well intended. It can be argued that he omitted women's opinions purposely, in order to elicit support for the female cause from men. Nevertheless, he perpetuated men's exclusion of the female voice from the public debate and legitimized the denial of female autonomy. However, as exemplified by Helene Lange and Käthe Schirmacher, many women claimed the voice denied to them. They did so on two levels: theoretically by writing in support of female education and practically by enrolling in universities.

2 Alleged Consequences of the Brain Structure and of the Anatomy of the Female Body

> *"Gehirn hin, Gehirn her!" sagte mein alter Professor, als ich mich mit ihm in einen Disput über die Frauenfrage eingelassen hatte. "Und wenn Sie mir hundertmal beweisen, daß das weibliche Gehirn im Verhältnis zur Körpergröße der Frau nicht kleiner ist, als das männliche, und daß kein Mikroskopiker im Stande war, einen Unterschied zwischen den Gehirnzellen und Gehirnfasern der Frau und denjenigen des Mannes zu entdecken, bleibe ich doch bei meinem alten, aus Erfahrung gewonnenen Sprichwort, daß Frauenzimmer lange Haare und kurzen Verstand haben."*
>
> Ludwig Büchner[98]

2.1 Introduction: Texts and Arguments Opening the Debates in Germany

Kirchhoff's survey was published in 1897 and presented a wide range of opinions regarding higher education for women at the very end of the nineteenth century. However, as indicated in the previous chapter, the public discussions about admission of women to the universities had started in Germany and Austria almost thirty years earlier, and by 1897 they had already changed their focus many times.[99] In the early 1860s, universities in the United States, Switzerland, and England allowed the first female students to participate in higher education. Admission of women to universities in these countries was looked upon by the rest of Europe as an experiment that would not bring positive results and would remain just an exception and not become a rule in higher education. However, approximately ten years later, admission of female students in Switzerland and England became an integral part of the educational policy in these countries. Moreover, progressive individuals demanded the same rights for women in other European countries, and higher education for women began to be taken more and more seriously. Although admission of women to German and Austrian universities was not even an option in 1860, by 1870 it was already considered a real possibility by many progressive individuals.[100] This fact seems to be the main motivation behind Theodor

98 Büchner 308.

99 Mazón divides the debate about admission of women to universities into two phases. According to her the debates in the 1870s focused on "contesting the legitimacy of the woman question," while the later debates were dominated by "the issues tied to academic citizenship" (113-114).

100 Precisely the readiness of many women to audit courses at various German universities was, according to Mazón, the cause for a general ban on women in late 1970s (Mazón 10; 119).

Bischoff's pamphlet *Das Studium und die Ausübung der Medizin durch Frauen*, in which he states: "[D]ie Zahl der Aerztinnen wächst; in Zürich studieren ihrer einige dreißig, in Edinburg zehn, an allen Universitäten machen sie den Versuch sich einzudrängen. Deshalb ist es nöthig, [...] daß man das ganze Unternehmen in seiner nackten und widerwärtigen Blöße darstellt" (39).

Bischoff, a professor of anatomy and physiology in Munich, published his pamphlet in 1872 with the intention to prove scientifically that women were not capable of studying medicine. He wanted to show that such an attempt would not only impair female health, but that it would also have a devastating impact on the entire medical profession. Bischoff was one of the first German academics who perceived women's entry into the public space of the university and science as a present danger and he published his brochure as a warning against it. *Das Studium und die Ausübung der Medizin durch Frauen* became a very popular text and elicited an abundance of positive and negative public responses. In the course of the debate about women's admission to medical schools, both opponents and supporters of the educational change referred to Bischoff's text numerous times.[101] Hence, I consider the year of the publication of Bischoff's pamphlet, 1872, the beginning of an intensive public resistance against female higher education in Germany. Two years later, Dohm responded to Bischoff by publishing *Die wissenschaftliche Emancipation der Frau.*[102] Her book constituted the first public female response to a specific text written by a male in the context of the struggle for women's admission to higher education at the end of the nineteenth century. The texts by Bischoff and Dohm denote only the first of several stages in the discussion surrounding admission of women to medical schools in Austria and Germany that I will discuss in the following chapters. However, I regard both texts as catalysts that propelled this debate on German ground during the following forty years.

2.2 The Female Brain

The desire to prove that the female brain is smaller than the male brain became a scientific obsession in the 1870s.[103] This fixation marked the brain as a typically male organ and thinking as a male domain. An equally well-developed brain in females was considered an anomaly. According to Schmersahl, comparative brain

101 Mazón confirms the popularity of Bischoff's theories. She quotes a university professor from Zurich, Arnold Dodel, who, reminiscing from a twenty-year perspective, verified Bischoff's authority at the time: "a word from his mouth or his pen was taken as the authoritative truth" (qtd. in Mazón 89). Mazón also claims that "[I]t was precisely the importance of Bischoff's book that later drove Dohm and others to respond to it" (89).

102 See also Mazón's discussion of Bischoff's text and Dohm's response to it (89-92).

103 See also Schmersahl 77 and the footnote 144 (77). Weiershausen emphasizes "die Bedeutung der Hirnforschung für die Geschlechterordnung, denn über sie wurde die behauptete geistige Verschiedenartigkeit der Geschlechter positivistisch *bewiesen*" (44). See also Weiershausen 44-45.

research that developed in the course of the nineteenth century was closely connected to the theory of evolution (76-77). It was Charles Darwin who provided a scientific foundation for the theories proclaiming women's inferiority by asserting that the physical and psychological differences between the sexes were results of different life tasks (Schmersahl 75-77). These tasks, in turn, required women to be passive and men active, meaning also "muthiger, kampflustiger und energischer" (Darwin qtd. in Schmersahl 76). As a result, as Schmersahl claims "war es möglich, den Mann als Subjekt des Evolutionsprozesses und damit als Träger von Fortschritt zu bestimmen" (76).

Among the scientists who worked on establishing a connection between brain size, gender, and intellectual development, Bischoff was best known for his findings. He examined 391 male and 253 female brains, comparing their weight and size, and concluded that because male brains were bigger and heavier, men were much better suited than women for any intellectual endeavors, in general, and for academic studies, in particular (Tichy, "Die geschlechtliche Un-Ordnung" 30). In his influential pamphlet Bischoff argued:

> Die Unterschiede in der Schädel- und Gehirnbildung [bei Frauen und Männern] sind so charakteristisch und wichtig, dass sie namentlich zur Beurtheilung der geistigen Unterschiede zwischen beiden Geschlechtern nicht übersehen werden dürfen. (15)

According to Bischoff, these differences had profound consequences as far as intellectual capabilities were concerned:

> Der männliche Geist sieht tiefer, weiter, schärfer, dringt mehr in das Innere der Dinge und berücksichtigt mehr das Wesen derselben, erforscht gründlicher und genauer, prüft ruhiger und urtheilt unbefangener. Der weibliche Geist berücksichtigt mehr das Aeussere, den Schein als das innere Wesen; sein Urtheil ist befangen, oberflächlich, sein Wille schwach, das Handeln unbestimmt. [...] Aus dieser Verschiedenartigkeit der Geschlechter in körperlicher und geistiger Hinsicht, geht unwiderleglich hervor, *dass das weibliche Geschlecht für das Studium und Pflege der Wissenschaften und insbesondere der Medicin nicht geeignet ist.* (20)

In her response to Bischoff, Dohm quoted the German scientist Reclam[104] who had researched the human brain extensively. According to Reclam (as paraphrased by Dohm) it was impossible to achieve any valid results regarding intellectual abilities by comparing male and female brains because

104 Reclam is not identified by his first name.

die Körperverhältnisse Beider [des Mannes und der Frau] [zeigen] zu bedeutende Abweichungen [...]. Man muß vielmehr die Hirngewichte eines und desselben Geschlechts mit einander [sic] vergleichen, was nur für Männergehirne ausführbar ist, da wir zu wenige Wägungen der Hirne geistig hochstehender Frauen besitzen. (*Emancipation* 88)

Dohm follows this line of argument by referring to many other scientists and anthropologists who refused to assess intellectual qualities based on the size of the human brain. By conducting extensive research on the issue and familiarizing herself with the scientific evidence of the time, Dohm was able to demonstrate that Bischoff's claims had at best equivalent, if not lesser, scientific value than the opposite convictions.

In 1883, Karl Bernhard Brühl[105] published an article entitled "Frauenhirn, Frauenseele, Frauenrecht," in which, according to the early feminists Mayreder and Binder, he disproved Bischoff's theory of the correlation between brain size and the intellectual potential of an individual (Mayreder, "Zur Physiologie" 68; Binder 13).[106] Brühl argued that such a complex organ could not be explored simply by weighing and measuring it, as Bischoff had suggested (Tichy, "Die geschlechtliche Un-Ordnung" 31). Additionally, Brühl discussed Bischoff's hypothesis extensively in two other texts: "Einiges über das Gehirn der Wirbelthiere mit besonderer Berücksichtigung jenes der Frau" (1879) and "Einiges über die Gaben der Natur an die Frau und die Konsequenzen hieraus für Bedeutung, Stellung, Aufgaben und Rechte der Frau in der menschlichen Gesellschaft. Eine anatomisch-soziologische Betrachtung mit Gehirn-Demonstration" (1892) (Sveistrup and v. Zahn-Harnack 6).[107]

By the 1890s, Bischoff's hypothesis was no longer taken seriously by most scientists. However, it is surprising to find that many opponents of women's education still referred to Bischoff as an expert on the issue at the end of the nineteenth century. It is rather obvious that the appeal of Bischoff's brain-size theory and its positive reception by opponents of female education had much more

105 See also Tichy, "Die geschlechtliche Un-Ordnung" 30-31; Schmersahl's footnote 146 (78).

106 Binder writes: "In einer eingehenden Studie, gestützt auf langjährige Forschung, lieferte der berühmte Anatom [Carl Bernhard Brühl] den Nachweis, daß die Lehre Bischoffs von der Gehirnbeschaffenheit des Weibes, samt den daraus gezogenen Schlüssen, vollständig unhaltbar und unverläßlich, und daß die Frau vermöge der Konstruktion ihres Gehirns zu wissenschaftlicher Arbeit nicht weniger befugt sei als der Mann. Er vertrat darin sogar die Ueberzeugung, daß eine entsprechende Behandlung des weiblichen Gehirns durch Erziehung, Unterricht, Einführung das Selbstvertrauen stärkender sozialer Verhältnisse und ähnliches, und durch eine hiermit auch naturhistorisch gegebene Weiterentwicklung der weiblichen Gehirnzellen, speziell ihres Großgehirns, zeigen werde, auch in der Neuzeit schon genügend gezeigt habe, daß das weibliche Gehirn ganz ungemein leistungsfähig sei, ja in manchen Leistungsbeziehungen sogar jenes des Mannes übertreffe" (13-14).

107 For other critical responses to Bischoff see Mazón 92-93.

to do with the theory's ideological underpinnings than with its scientific validity.[108] Binder underlines the ideological appeal that Bischoff's theory had for many:

> Daß er [Bischoff] selbst bei Begründung seiner Sätze sonderbarerweise gar keinen Wert darauf legte erstens, daß es Tiere giebt, deren Gehirn um zwei Drittel schwerer wiegt als jedes Männergehirn, und zweitens, daß das relative Hirngewicht, d.h. das Hirngewicht im Verhältnis zum Körpergewicht zu Gunsten der Frau sich verhält, genierte vorderhand nur wenige. Die dünkelhafte Anmaßung der Weiber schien wieder einmal gründlich ad absurdum geführt und darüber war Freude auf allen Gassen. (12-13)

Mayreder summarizes the entire brain debate and writes about its impact on women's demands for higher education in her article "Zur Physiologie des weiblichen Geschlechtes" published in *Dokumente der Frauen* in April 1899. She points out that Bischoff's theory regarding female inferiority, based on the size of the brain, enjoyed positive publicity for a fairly long time (Mayreder 67). She also shows that the seemingly obvious counter-arguments, such as the considerable brain size of many animals, the relative weight of the brain, and the lack of correlation between the brain mass and the intellectual potential, did not seem to enter the debate on the side of the opponents of female higher education. Studies of the brain size in animals never demonstrated anything about intelligence as the human-based studies were trying to do. A witty and sharp writer, Mayreder ridicules Bischoff's theory as follows:

> Sattsam bekannt ist der Fall Bischoff, jenes Münchener Professors, der die Lehre von dem geringeren Gehirngewicht des Weibes in die Welt setzte, eine Lehre, die durch eine Laune der Natur ironisiert wurde; denn es stellte sich nach seinem Tode heraus, dass sein Gehirn noch um 5 Gramm weniger wog, als das Durchschnittsgewicht des weiblichen Gehirnes nach seiner Angabe betragen sollte. ("Zur Physiologie" 67)

The fact that Bischoff's hypothesis was officially disproved did not discourage other medical scientists from looking for evidence of the alleged female intellectual inferiority in the brain.[109] Nicolaus Rüdinger, too, tried to prove it by weighing and measuring brains. He followed Bischoff's example by comparing the brains of twins. The brain of the boy turned out to be further developed than the brain of the girl, and this was a sufficient proof for Rüdinger to generalize about female inferiority (Tichy, "Die geschlechtliche Un-Ordnung" 31). Havelock

108 See also Mazón 93.
109 See also Schmersahl 78.

Ellis, an English physician and advocate of women's rights, argued against both Bischoff and Rüdinger in his book *Man and Woman: a Study of Human Secondary Sexual Characters* that was first published in 1894. In an article, "Das Gehirn der Frauen," published in *Die Zukunft*, he explained that studies following Rüdinger's research delivered different results. The difference in the brain weight between newborn boys and girls turned out to be much smaller than Rüdinger had claimed. In addition, Ellis pointed out that

> [u]nter den Neugeborenen, die auf den Seeziertisch kommen, finden sich mehr Knaben mit großen Köpfen, weil ungewöhnlich große Köpfe bei Knaben häufiger als bei Mädchen sind und dementsprechend auch die Todesfälle bei der Geburt; diese Ausnahmefälle beeinflussen das Resultat der Hirnwägungen Neugeborener im Sinne eines größeren männlichen Durchschnittsgewicht. (132)

After the scientific community stopped taking the theories based on the brain's size and weight seriously, some scientists and physicians attempted to show that particular parts of the brain display structural and developmental differences between men and women. The issue proved controversial. In 1877 Rüdinger found out that the parietal lobe exhibited a more intensive development in male brains, and his student Passet confirmed these results in 1882 (Ellis 133). Binder depicted these findings as a second phase in the attempts to discredit women's cognitive ability based on the structure of her brain:

> Seit diesen Ausführungen Brühls sind acht Jahre vergangen und auch der verbissenste Gehirnwäger ist stumm geworden. Dafür kamen die Gegner des Frauenstudiums nunmehr mit einem Scheitellappen herangezogen, der beim Manne angeblich stärker oder anders gefurcht sein soll als beim Weibe, und stellten sich als glaubten sie, daß hierdurch das männliche Gehirn vor dem weiblichen etwas voraus habe. (14)

Ellis showed that Rüdinger's and Passet's findings regarding the development of the parietal lobe were scientifically not acceptable because the number of brains used in the experiments was too small, and because it was very difficult to examine the brain due to its high level of variability (133). In addition, Ellis contended that there was no proven connection between the parietal lobe and intellect. Finally, he asserted:

> Man kann kaum sagen, daß der gegenwärtige Standpunkt der Hirnforschung irgend welche wichtigen Geschlechtsunterschiede aufgedeckt hätte. Künftig, wenn die Thatsachen genauer festgestellt sind und ihre Bedeutung verständlicher ist, wird Das [sic] vielleicht

anders sein. Heute muß man die Thatsache betonen, daß die Bedeutung des Gehirns für das Problem der Geschlechtsunterschiede sehr übertrieben worden ist. (Ellis 136)

Tichy quotes other scientists of the nineteenth century who, like Ellis, rejected brain experiments and concludes that procedures used by Bischoff and Rüdinger were not considered scientific even at the time ("Die geschlechtliche Un-Ordnung" 31). As Kirchhoff's survey demonstrates, by the 1890s at the latest, "brain proofs" were discredited by the majority of the scientific community.

However, when a number of professors of medicine (Karl von Bardeleben, Isidor Rosenthal, and Ottomar Rosenbach among others) rejected "brain proofs" as scientifically unacceptable (Kirchhoff 33; 54; 82), it was only the methods of scientific inquiry that they questioned, not the actual findings. In other words, it was not so much female inferiority and inability to pursue an academic education that were questioned, but the causal relationship between brain size and intellectual abilities. This conviction, in turn, was ridiculed in an article, "Das Gehirn der Frau," written by Ludwig Büchner for the progressive journal *Die Frau* in February 1894, from which I chose a paragraph as a motto for this chapter. As indicated by this passage, many opponents of women's education took the notion of woman's intellectual inferiority for granted and refused to renounce this belief even in the absence of scientific proof. Büchner also hints at the fact that the perception of female inferiority is so deeply rooted in the popular understanding of gender differences that it would take much more than scientific proof to change it. In the anecdote, the old professor uses a misogynistic proverb to justify his conviction of female intellectual inferiority because it suits his views better than scientific evidence. By doing so, he refuses to imagine an alternative social order.

2.3 The Correlation between (Pseudo) Scientific Pamphlets and Political Decisions

During the meeting of German scientists and physicians in Cologne in Fall 1888, privy councilor (Geheimrat) and professor of medicine Wilhelm Waldeyer gave a speech entitled "Das Studium der Medicin und die Frauen" that was subsequently published in the September edition of *Tagesblatt der Versammlung Deutscher Naturforscher und Ärzte*.[110] Waldeyer was not only very sympathetic towards Bischoff as a colleague,[111] but he was also like-minded in his opinions regarding female medical education. Therefore, in his speech he warned against women's admission to medical schools, which he perceived as a profoundly negative influence not only on the development of medical sciences but also on the whole

110 Mazón contends that Waldeyer's speech was a response to Mathilde Weber's pamphlet, *Ärztinnen für Frauenkrankheiten* (108). For a discussion of Waldeyer's arguments and Morgenstern's response to him see also Mazón 108-112.

111 Waldeyer refers to Bischoff as to "meinem hochverehrten verstorbenen Kollegen" 40.

human race. In addition it would have negative consequences for women themselves (Waldeyer 37).

In his speech, Waldeyer refers to both Bischoff and Rüdinger as scientific authorities and recalls their brain research, although he admits that Bischoff might indeed have been slightly blinded by his hostility towards women's emancipation (40). He emphasizes throughout his speech that women were never able to achieve at the same intellectual and creative level as men. He writes: "[B]is zu dem Niveau, welches die Männer erreichten, haben sie [Frauen] sich nicht erhoben. Das kann keine äusseren Gründe haben, das ist in der natürlichen Organisation des Weibes tief gewurzelt" (Waldeyer 39). Although Waldeyer is careful enough to state that physical differences do not provide sufficient evidence of female intellectual inferiority, ["Wollen wir wohl beachten, dass ich aus diesen körperlichen Verschiedenheiten keine Schlüsse ziehe auf eine etwaige *Unterordnung* des Weibes in geistiger Beziehung" (40)], he nonetheless claims: "Aber das ist richtig, dass die Beanlagung des Mannes ihn mehr befähigt, eine Wissenschaft und Kunst höher zu treiben und rascher zu fördern" (40). To provide evidence, he refers his audience to the histories of art and science. Waldeyer's argumentation very closely resembles the logic of the old professor in Ludwig Büchner's article. It is apparent that Waldeyer does not base his conviction of female intellectual inferiority on scientific research. On the contrary, it seems to be rooted in prejudice and tradition, forces that, according to Dohm, created and sustained female subjugation.

Weber connects the failure of the 1888 petition to "Unterrichts-Ministerien verschiedener deutschsprachiger Staaten" (4) regarding women's admission to medical schools[112] with Waldeyer's speech for two reasons. As privy councilor, Waldeyer was a well-known and respected personality, and by virtue of speaking publicly against female medical education he made his animosity against women known to a wider audience (Weber 5).[113] Lange, too, points to Waldeyer's influence on the matter of female medical education (*Frauenbildung* 88). By using his political influence to propagate personal misogynistic views, Waldeyer was able, consciously or not, to sabotage women's attempt to gain access to medical education. Weber explains Waldeyer's negative influence on the woman's question as follows:

---

112 According to Glaser, Weber's pamphlet, *Ärztinnen für Frauenkrankheiten*, accompanied the 1888 petition "an die Regierung der Einzelstaaten" ("Die erste Studentinnengeneration" 312). See also Mazón 74.

113 Glaser hints at the corellation between the medical and political spheres: "Festgehalten werden muß, daß die Gegner des Frauenstudiums in den meisten Fällen Mitglieder der medizinischen Fakultäten waren und in den Standesorganisationen wichtige Funktionen innehatten" ("Die erste Studentinnengeneration" 318). Mazón explicitely restates this connection: "[T]he power and influence of the individual professor were not limited to his classroom but could reach the state education ministry through faculty and senate votes on important issues" (86) For the secondary literature on this issue see Mazón's footnote 3 (86; 245).

> Die große Menge, welche nicht gerne selbst denkt und prüft, hat eine entscheidende Neigung zur blinden Nachbetung des Ausspruches einer Autorität. Auch die gegnerische Presse bemächtigte sich mit Schadenfreude dieser Angriffe gegen unsere Wünsche um Frauenärztinnen; so konnten damals diejenigen maßgebenden Behörden [...] die Erhörung unserer Bitten bequem wieder hinausschieben. (5)

Weber refers to the situation in 1888, the year in which the fourth edition of her text was published. However, in the introduction to the fifth edition of her book issued in 1893, she can reflect on Waldeyer's influence from a five-year distance. She pointed out that the situation in 1893 was much more favorable to women's struggle for admission to medical schools. Based on the support of the issue expressed by Karl Baumbach, chief mayor of Danzig and vice president of the German parliament, in his speech on February 23, 1893, Weber could be more sanguine regarding the official decision in this matter. She states: "Alle Anzeigen bürgen uns dafür, daß diese Petition mit mehr Wohlwollen und mehr Zugeständnis an den Zeitgeist behandelt werden wird, als die frühere, welche unter dem Banne von Geheimrat Waldeyers feindlicher Rede gelitten hatte" (Weber 5). Weber stresses the influence that the public debates exerted on legislation regarding this matter.[114] Obviously, the support for or the opposition to admission of women to medical schools on the part of politically influential personalities had a direct impact on legislative decisions. Yet the influence of the progressive female voice in public discussions should not be underestimated.[115]

2.4 Other Anatomical Differences

As already demonstrated, Bischoff was not alone in claiming the superiority of the male. In fact, this theory was quite fashionable and, as Mazón pointed out,

---

114 For a discussion of petitions to German authorities issued by various women's organizations see Glaser, "Die erste Studentinnengeneration" 314-18; Mazón 59-60; 70-72; 74; 78-79; 97.

115 Mazón referrs to Albisetti who emphasized "the success with the *Frauenstudium* as one of the main achievements of the German middle-class women's movement" (12) and who "has noted, petitions were unsuccessful in parliament but stimulated public discussion nonetheless" (97). Burchardt points out that in the course of the following twenty years Waldeyer changed his attitude towards medical education for women: "Der Berliner Anatom Waldeyer, der sich 1888 noch als entschiedener Gegner des Frauenmedizinstudiums gezeigt hatte, hatte seine Meinung im Laufe der folgenden 20 Jahre geändert, er stand nun einem Universitätsstudium der Frauen nicht mehr ablehnend gegenüber. Er beharrte jedoch weiterhin auf seiner Forderung nach gesonderten Frauenuniversitäten. Selbst nach Zulassung zur regulären Immatrikulation für Frauen weigerte Waldeyer sich, männliche und weibliche Studenten gemeinsam zu unterrichten, und ließ statt dessen von einem seiner Assistenten in der Dachkammer des Berliner Anatomischen Instituts einen gesonderten Anatomiekurs für Studentinnen abhalten" (16-17). For Waldeyer's change of opinion in regard to higher education for women see also Mazón 112.

"Bischoff's argument about female inferiority represented the latest medical research at the time" (94-95). In addition to citing the theory of the underdeveloped brain in females, Bischoff centers his argument against higher education for women on the premise that there are profound anatomical differences between males and females and "dass sich diese Verschiedenheiten nicht etwa nur auf einige Unterschiede in den äußersten Formen und den Geschlechtsorganen, sondern [...] auf jeden Knochen, jeden Muskel, jedes Organ, jeden Nerven, jede Faser erstrecken" (14). These disparities, in turn, determine the abilities, character, and personality traits of all individuals. Hence, women are in every regard different from men and are not able to achieve what men can. These gender-specific characteristics create a relationship of natural inequality between men and women, with men being superior to women. Bischoff argues that "das Weib entschieden ungleich schwächer ist, in seiner Organisation einen minder hohen Entwicklungsgrad erreicht hat, und in allen Beziehungen dem Kinde näher steht, als der Mann" (14). Again, Bischoff was not the only one who saw substantial similarities between women and children. This connection, although also broadened to incorporate people of other races and animals in addition to women and children, had been part of Western thinking on gender and other differences.[116] Schmersahl argues, it was "als Denkmodell an sich nicht neu" (83), but what was really new was the "scientific" foundation of these theories, made possible by Darwin's findings (Schmersahl 83). In addition, as Schmersahl writes, "Darwin's 1871 entwickelte Theorie der 'sexuellen Zuchtwahl' beruhte auf der Annahme, daß die Geschlechterdifferenz ein integraler Bestandteil des Evolutionsprozesses sei" (84).[117] Even though he was most likely familiar with Darwin's theory, Bischoff drew similar conclusions from his own research.[118]

Although Bischoff's main intent was to prove that the female brain is less developed than the male and therefore is not capable of the same intellectual work, in the appendix to his pamphlet, he provides a very specific anatomical description not only of the skull and brain but also of the internal and external male and female body characteristics. The fixation on gender differences gives the impression that he is analyzing two completely different and incompatible species rather than beings of the same species.[119] Dohm points out in her article "Die Ritter der *mater dolorosa*" that this frequently employed argument of female "Anderswertigkeit" has obviously negative and dangerous implications. It relegates women to an inferior position and almost equates woman and animal: "Das Tier ist auch in

116 Runge and Möbius, discussed later in this book, made the same connection.

117 For a discussion of Darwin's theories used both in support of and in opposition to women's emancipation see Schmersahl 74-83.

118 Schmersahl emphasizes the reciprocal connection between the theory of evolution and the research of human brain and anatomy during the nineteenth century 78.

119 It is important to keep in mind that Bischoff's argument is undermined by the class to which he belongs. Dohm's critique of his lack of class-consciousness will be discussed later in this chapter.

seinem Beruf und seiner Art nur anderswertig, nicht minderwertig, als der Mensch" (34). This statement brings to mind a novel by Helene Böhlau entitled *Halbtier. Ein Frauenroman,* published in 1899; its title refers to the status of women in German society.

Bischoff sees man and woman as two opposites with strictly assigned roles in society that are not an object of negotiation. Gender roles are derived from anatomical structures of the human body; they are determined by nature and therefore should not be changed. Any change would be a violation of the laws of nature resulting in pathological effects, to which Bischoff refers as an inevitable "Strafe der Natur" (22). The division of labor and a gender-specific assignment of particular life domains are results of the anatomical differences between men and women. Higher education and especially the study of medicine are reserved exclusively for men because the female body is not suited for such pursuits.

Dohm opposes such a deterministic gender theory and relegates it to the position of a hypothesis that cannot be scientifically proven. According to her, gender roles are the consequences of centuries of oppression and of physical force. Hence, they are negotiable and changeable. She shows that Bischoff's methods of scientific inquiry do not fulfill scientific criteria. In addition to proceeding unscientifically ("unwissenschaftlich"), he presents his results in an insincere ("nicht redlich") way:

> Unwissenschaftlich, denn er läßt sich zu einer phrenologischen Lokalisierung der Seelenkräfte verleiten, während unsere Unkenntnis der Naturgesetze in Bezug auf die Spezialverrichtungen des Gehirns und der Umstände, unter denen es sich entwickelt, zweifellos ist. [...] Herr v. Bischof [sic] verfährt nicht redlich, indem er uns nur die Resultate derjenigen Untersuchungen vorlegt, die seinen Vorurtheilen entsprechen, die ihnen widersprechenden aber ignoriert. (*Emancipation* 86)

Dohm argues that Bischoff's theories of female inferiority based on the anatomical differences between the sexes are only "willkürliche Hypothesen" (*Emancipation* 86) without any scientific value. She points out that variations of the bodily structure between men and women do not prove female inferiority; she refers to another scientist, the French physiologist Tussenel,[120] who, on the basis of the same anatomical differences argued exactly the opposite–female superiority (*Emancipation* 86-87). Referring to the (pseudo) scientific research that attempts to disqualify women's demands, Mayreder, too, points out that such research is not reliable, especially with regard to the interpretation of its findings ("Die Physiologie" 68).

120 Dohm does not identify him by his first name.

2.5 Gender-Specific Division of Labor

According to both Bischoff and Waldeyer, women are not able to fulfill the same tasks as men on the basis of different anatomic and mental qualities, which results in a gender-specific and natural division of labor. In *Das Studium und die Ausübung der Medicin durch Frauen*, Bischoff contends that "Frauen Das [sic] nicht leisten können, was Männer vermögen, sowie umgekehrt diese nicht, was Jene" (14). For him, as for most opponents of female education, all occupations are "assigned" to men and women by nature, therefore all occupations are biologically determined.[121] In her response, Dohm asserts that there is no biologically determined and natural division of labor. Women are able to carry out the same type of work as men. In case of very difficult and physically draining work, for example in factories and mines, women perform exactly the same tasks as men, and they are not kept from this inhumane labor on the basis of their "delicate" constitution. Instead, women are barred from lucrative jobs. Therefore, she concludes, mere economic factors with a built-in male power structure determine this separation of the professional work force along gender lines: "die geistige Arbeit und die einträgliche für die Männer, die mechanische und die schlecht bezahlte Arbeit für die Frauen" (*Emancipation* 11).

Although Dohm is aware of the inhumane working conditions for both men and women in mines and factories, she provides statistical evidence to show that women are treated worse and earn much less money than men for the same type of physical labor. According to Dohm, the main reason for paying low wages to blue-collar female workers is their lack of the professional instruction that men receive. The glove-making industry, for instance, employs both male and female workers, but men earn twice as much as women: "Der Mangel professioneller Ausbildung macht sie [Frauen] unfähig für das Zuschneiden und Glätten der Handschuhe. Nur das Nähen, Steppen und Sticken bleibt ihnen überlassen" (*Emancipation* 17). Dohm concludes: "In allen Gewerben, welche Kenntnisse und eine gründliche Lehrzeit erfordern, sind die Frauen untergeordnet, in den ungesunden Gewerben dagegen, welche kurze Lehrzeit beanspruchen, herrschen sie vor" (*Emancipation* 18). Working-class women are kept from professional instruction in the same way as middle-class women are excluded from universities. In other words, any kind of education that qualifies an individual for a better-paying job is inaccessible to women and remains in Germany only a male domain. Middle-class women are kept from any type of professional work with the same determination with which working-class women are forced into low-wage, inhumane physical labor.

---

121 Schmersahl argues that scientific theories about the alleged female otherness conveniently supported work division within bourgeois society. She writes: "Die aufmerksame Lektüre der sexualwissenschaftlichen Literatur macht deutlich, wie sehr die Definition einer angeblich naturgebenen 'weiblichen' Sexualität und die aus dieser abgeleitete Stellung der Frau sich letztendlich aus den Erfordernissen einer arbeitsteilig organisierten bürgerlichen Gesellschaft ergaben" (72).

In both cases women are completely dependent on a male provider. Dohm implies that working-class women are not able to survive on their low wages, and their income must be supplemented by that of their husbands in order to provide adequately for the family. Similarly, middle-class women do not have access to any source of income and are in most cases totally dependent on their husbands. Middle-class single women and widows are often forced to take on blue-collar jobs for which they are not prepared and end up on the street or dead. Women could avoid such a fate if they had not been brought up to be dependent on men, but such an alternative was not available to them. It is irresponsible to train women to be wives without preparing them for an alternative: "Die Frauen werden zur Abhängigkeit erzogen; ob sich aber in der Noth des Lebens Jemand findet, von dem sie abhängen, darum bekümmert man sich nicht!" (Dohm, *Emancipation* 23). Dependency on others is not an innate quality in the case of women, as Bischoff believes, but is produced through social norms and values. Therefore, it is possible for women to become self-reliant and independent if they receive appropriate schooling. Education and work training would grant better jobs for women which, in turn, would lead to their financial independence. Women would not have to depend on marriage as a means for survival, and different gender relations would be the result. In Dohm's opinion men fight against the admission of women to higher education because it could result in a rearrangement of the social order and in males being less privileged. Dohm provides specific examples to show that this fear of female competition exists mainly among middle-class men:

> Ein Beweis dafür ist der Umstand, daß jeder Mann das unermeßlich wichtige Geschäft, das er gerade betreibt, für denjenigen Beruf hält, den auszufüllen Gott und die Natur der Frau versagt haben. Herr v. Bischof [sic] glaubt, daß die Frau alles Andere eher leisten könne, als die Ausübung der Medicin. Unter den schädlichen Folgen der medicinischen Studien der Frauen hebt er hervor: "die unausbleibliche Verdrängung männlicher Ärzte." Er giebt aber den Frauen seinen Segen für irgend welche Beschäftigung beim Post- und Telegraphendienst, und die unausbleibliche Verdrängung männlicher Postbeamten vergißt er dabei. Der Herr General-Postdirektor Stephan dagegen ist der Ansicht, daß die Frau zu allem Anderen eher geeignet sei, als zum Postdienst. Wiederum Professor v. Sybel behauptet, sie könne eher Medicin studieren, als irgend eine andere Wissenschaft. (*Emancipation* 25-26)

It is clear from this passage that decisions to exclude women from specific academic disciplines were motivated by the desire to favor men in the various professions. The benefit of women does not appear to be a real concern. Hence, as most of the female writers indicated, women were just second-class citizens whose lives had only a secondary value.

Like Bischoff, Waldeyer also insists on a gender specific division of labor. He resists women's attempts to gain access to the medical profession based on two principles: "das Prinzip der Arbeitstheilung" and "die Zweigeschlechtlichkeit des Menschenstammes" (Waldeyer 42). Waldeyer argues that the first principle is a natural rule that not only humans but also animals have to obey. Hence, it is not socially constructed but imposed by nature on all living beings. The second principle is irreversibly connected to the first one:

> Die Vertheilung der Menschheit auf zwei Geschlechter, von denen jedes mit besonderen Gaben und Fähigkeiten ausgerüstet, mit besonderen Neigungen behaftet ist, stellt eine der grossartigsten Arbeitstheilungen vor und wird als solche dem Ganzen nutzbar, wenn jeder Theil die ihm von der Natur zugewiesenen Aufgaben innerhalb ihrer Grenzen getreu kultiviert. (Waldeyer 42-43)

According to Waldeyer, women's entrance into the medical profession would constitute a transgression of the natural principle of the division of labor and consequently could lead to the erasure of gender differences. Such a process, however, would mean the deterioration of the human race because the main characteristic of highly developed species is a profound difference between both sexes.[122]

Weber,[123] less radical than Dohm,[124] agrees with Waldeyer as far as the natural gender-specific division of labor is concerned, but she modifies his classification by adding a gender-neutral work field to the typically male and female ones. She contends that both men and women can work successfully in any gender-neutral professional area without jeopardizing their gender characteristics. According to her, medicine is one example of such a neutral discipline (Weber 7). She even singles out the medical profession as a natural call for women:

> Neigung und Verständnis, sowie jener Drang der Natur, auf den die Gegner einen so großen Wert legen, ist zu tief in der zum Helfen stets bereiten Frauenbrust eingewurzelt. – Es ist auch erst in diesem Jahrhundert den Gegnern möglich geworden, diesen unaustilgbaren Hang der Frauen zur Heilkunde der Gesellschaft als falsches Emanzipations-gelüste darzustellen. (Weber 7)

Weber clearly believes in specific gender-based characteristics, but precisely because of this conviction, she demands the opening of medical schools to German women. At the same time, she is aware that the opponents of medical education

122 See also the discussion of Darwin and the reception of the theory of evolution in Schmersahl 84.

123 See also Mazón's summary of Lange's (74-76; 82) and Weber's arguments (80-81).

124 Mazón points out that "Dohm's views are often characterized as the most individualist and liberal articulated by anyone associated with the women's movement" (56).

for women have manipulated public opinion into believing in the unnatural or even perverted nature of these demands by distorting reality. Weber points out that the demand for medical education is not just a female whim but a call of nature and a social necessity: "[D]as 'Doktorieren' geht nicht aus Emanzipationslust, sondern gerade aus den weiblichen Eigenschaften hervor und geschieht vielfach aus augenblicklicher Notwendigkeit" (8).

Similarly, Lange agrees with Waldeyer on the issue of the natural gender-specific division of labor and admits that women should indeed remain in the realm that suits their nature and development.[125] However, she challenges his notion of a kind of specifically female labor by indicating that it is man, not nature, who sets social standards. Lange points her finger at the male dominance in society and argues that men suppress the natural female call to the medical profession for the sake of their own advantages. Thus, she sees the female struggle for admission to medical schools as "ein Kampf der Natur gegen die, die sie unterdrücken wollen" (*Frauenbildung* 91). Although she admits that men and women have different roles in society, she rejects Waldeyer's claim that these differences can or should be translated into a separation of professional occupations:

> Die notwendige Arbeitsteilung scheint mir durchaus nicht mit der von Professor Waldeyer so plausibel gemachten Berufsteilung zusammenzufallen. Da hätten jedenfalls wir Frauen noch recht viel zu fordern, denn die Berufe gehören fast alle den Männern. [...] Die innere Leitung des Hauswesens, das stille Walten in der Familie wird sich die Frau nie nehmen lassen; die Verteidigung dieses Hausfriedens nach außen durch physische Kraft wird sich der Mann vorbehalten. In dieser Trennung liegt Natur; nicht aber in der Trennung von geistiger und mechanischer Arbeit, von denen letztere willig, auch wo sie große physische Anstrengung erfordert, der Frau zuerkannt, erstere als die interessantere, befriedigendere und – lohnendere vom Manne reklamiert wird. Die Frauen haben dasselbe Recht auf geistige Arbeit wie der Mann, und die Differenzierung der Geschlechter wird immer nur zum Teil in der Berufsteilung zum Ausdruck kommen. (*Frauenbildung* 91-92)

125 Mazón sees Weber's and Lange's views of femininity and the role they should play in professional life as quite similar (74; 81-82). Both women "offered reassurances about gender roles, insisting that education would enhance womanly values, not erode them" (Mazón 82). Both also emphasized that women should be admitted to the medical profession because of their "nurturing qualities" (Mazón 82) and the special contribution they would bring into the medical field on the basis of their "otherness" (76; 82). In addition, Weber and Lange used the rhetoric of "service for other women" in their arguments (Mazón 75; 81). See also Mazón's summary of Lange's (74-76; 82) and Weber's arguments (80-81).

Lange believes in a natural distribution of certain tasks in life between males and females. Following the traditional understanding of gender roles, she attributes emotional caring for the family to women and its physical protection to men. It is clear that, unlike Dohm, Lange does not question the notion of innate gender characteristics. However, she refuses to assign intellectual qualities only to one sex. As suggested in the quoted passage, Lange distinguishes three dimensions of a human being: physical, emotional, and intellectual. While she recognizes a clear split between the physical and the emotional realms along gender lines, she perceives the intellectual dimension as having the potential to be equally developed in both sexes. By doing so, she redefines what are believed to be traditional gendered qualities. She shows that the natural division of tasks in the family does not predispose women to physical and men to intellectual work. On the contrary, men who usually display greater physical force should be naturally responsible for mechanical labor. However, in the middle and upper classes, the opposite is the case as Binder ironically points out in an every-day scenario in which a middle- and upper-class man feels it necessary "nach dem Dienstmädchen zu rufen, wenn etwa ein Kasten zu rücken, oder ein gefüllter Handkoffer vom Fußboden auf den Tisch zu heben ist" (20).

As stated by Lange, women are allowed to perform only physical work, whereas men have access to all professions in German society. The conclusion is obvious. While for Lange there is a natural gender-specific division of tasks in the family, professional life involving material profit is controlled by men not by virtue of nature but because of male dominance in society. Lange argues that precisely because of the differences between the sexes, certain professions would benefit from being open to both men and women (*Frauenbildung* 92). Since, according to Lange, there are gender-specific characteristics and personality traits, each of the sexes would be able to contribute to and enrich their profession in a different way. Therefore, the medical profession would only profit from a female presence, especially with regard to such disciplines as gynecology, obstetrics, and pediatrics.

2.6 Class and Gender

While Bischoff and Waldeyer focus exclusively on sex and gender, women participating in the discussion about higher education point to the importance of class and social status in this debate. Binder and Lange argue that gender characteristics of individuals are modified according to class. Thus, they confirm Dohm's claim that it is the work done by an individual that influences his/her gender-specific qualities. Although not articulated explicitly by these women, it is very clear that they, unlike Bischoff and Waldeyer, differentiate between sex and gender. According to Binder and Lange, gender differences are much more noticeable in the upper and middle classes, while they almost seem to disappear in the working class. Consequently, they argue, Waldeyer's "Prinzip der Arbeitstheilung" and "die Zweigeschlechtlichkeit des Menschenstammes" are at work to a much greater degree in the upper and middle classes. In the higher social classes gender differences are sustained artificially through upbringing and gender-specific education. Binder quotes Theobald Ziegler on the issue of gender differences in the upper and middle classes: "In den oberen Schichten unseres Volkes, wo die beiden Geschlechter in ganz verschiedener Weise erzogen werden, Mann und Weib beinahe kein gemeinsames Arbeitsgebiet haben, erscheint jene Differenz [d.h. der geistige Unterschied] nach und nach in geradezu schädlicher Weise künstlich erweitert und gespannt" (Binder 15). Intellectual differences between men and women are then not natural, but are maintained artificially. While men are encouraged to pursue academic endeavors, women are discouraged from such a pursuit regardless of their intellectual potential. Additionally, there is no common working environment for men and women that would allow both sexes to develop similar skills or qualifications because middle-class men work mainly in liberal professions while their wives stay at home and are not gainfully employed. Such a division of tasks and labor is profitable to men but harmful to women because they cannot be financially independent. Binder argues:

> Schulung und Bildung der beiden Geschlechter [in den oberen Schichten der Bevölkerung, im sogennanten höheren Mittelstand] in getrennten, und zwar nach Art und Ziel völlig getrennten Bahnen laufend, die Frau thatsächlich und von rechtswegen ausgeschlossen von beinahe allen Arbeits- und Erwerbsgebieten, bloß, weil der Mann sie inne hat, fehlerhaft entwickelt darum an Thatkraft und Lebensgeschicklichkeit, nach jeder Richtung verhindert, sich auf die eigenen Füße zu stellen, und doch hierzu durch die Gesamtheit der Verhältnisse, namentlich auch die fort- schreitende Verarmung der besseren Klassen, so häufig und so dringend verpflichtet. (3)

The middle-class woman is destined to be financially dependent on her husband and consciously prepared by her parents for a life without any possibility for autonomy. In addition, through such an upbringing, she is formed to be the exact opposite of men as far as personality traits, character, and the level of knowledge are concerned because the female appeal is believed to be derived precisely from these differences. In this context, Lange also emphasizes that gender differences in the upper and middle classes are created artificially: "Ein *willkürlich* geschaffenes, also auch leicht abzustellendes Mißverhältnis besteht erst in den mittleren und oberen Klassen [...]. Hier erst steht der Mann der Frau privilegiert gegenüber; er hat außer den Vorteilen, die die Natur ihm verlieh, noch eine Menge von Vorteilen, die ihm die Gesellschaft, d.h. er selbst, zugesprochen hat" (*Frauenbildung* 86). According to Lange, unlike in the lower classes the differences in privileges between men and women in the upper classes are very significant. Natural advantages men have in life are magnified and complemented by the ones that are not innate, but artificially created. The women's movement aimed at the elimination of socially created rights that grant men all possible concessions at the cost of women's freedom and autonomy.

Dohm calls attention to a contradiction present in male arguments regarding gender differences. On the one hand, opponents of female medical education claim that there are profound natural differences in body structure, personality traits, and other characteristics between men and women. On the other hand, however, they also argue that a woman's intellectual development could potentially eliminate some of these differences. Dohm comes to the following conclusion:

> Die Männer scheinen anzunehmen, daß nicht die schöpferische Kraft der Natur den Geschlechtern die Verschiedenheit eingebildet habe (in diesem Falle wäre sie ja unaustilgbar), sondern daß dieselbe erst künstlich entwickelt werden müßte, und darum lautet ihr Verdikt: "Lasset die Knäblein Griechisch lernen und Lateinisch und Mathematik u.s.w. Die Mägdlein aber lasset nicht Griechisch, nicht Lateinisch und nicht Mathematik lernen, damit die Verschiedenheit der Geschlechter herrlich wachse und gedeihe!" (*Emancipation* 177-178)

According to Binder and Lange, the situation of working-class women is entirely different. There is no real division of labor along gender lines because women are forced to take on the same difficult and physically draining jobs as men. They share "Arbeitsgebiet, Erwerbsrecht und Erwerbspflicht" (Binder 3) equally. In this class, neither men nor women receive education and, as adults, neither have developed intellectually. Therefore, both sexes are equally prepared for the existential struggle. Lange also contends that unlike in the upper and middle classes, in the working class there are no artificially created differences between the sexes. She claims that lower-class women are able to find a job relatively easily and enjoy equality with men. Although, she admits, many women have to struggle with poverty and very difficult living and working conditions, they are in the same situation as men. Lange sees the woman's question as being specific to the higher classes and seems to sympathize much more with these women. She distances herself from the woman's question of the lower classes because she perceives it as an integral part of a more general social question: "Die Frauenfrage in den unteren Ständen macht [...] nur einen integrierenden Teil der sozialen Frage aus und hängt mit ihrer Lösung zusammen" (*Frauenbildung* 86).

Lange makes a clear distinction between two class-specific sources of women's subjugation. She points out that while the existence of lower-class women is usually wretched by virtue of their economic status, the life of middle-class women is made miserable by virtue of their sex. In the lower classes women share oppression with men. In the upper classes only women lack freedom and agency by virtue of having been turned into objects of male pleasure and into commodities. However, she admits that although female lives in different social classes have always been determined by diverse factors, they also exhibited a certain resemblance, namely, regardless of their social status, women have always been objectified and de-personalized: "Sie [die Frau] ist entweder Sklavin oder Luxusartikel gewesen" (*Frauenbildung* 88). In contrast, Dohm claims that even among the working class, men enjoy a much more privileged position than women by virtue of their gender.

Dohm notes the virtual exclusion of lower-class women from Bischoff's category "female" and makes us aware of the intersections between class and gender. Working-class women seem to lack "typical feminine traits" such as "zarte Konstitution" and "Schamhaftigkeit" because otherwise they would not be able to work in mines and factories (*Emancipation* 12). Although Bischoff claims to write about women in general, he only draws a caricature of bourgeois women. Dohm confronts this unrealistic representation of femininity with a more authentic image of working-class women and shows that both the representation and reality are completely distinct. By doing so, she redefines Bischoff's narrow and simplistic notion of femininity. Dohm asserts that occupation, upbringing, and a way of living influence the character and personality traits of a person in a much more profound way than anatomy and biological sex (*Emancipation* 83). A female bar owner is most likely anything but humble, submissive, and gentle (*Emancipation* 84) because otherwise she would not be able to maintain her business. Her characteristics are a result of her social status and occupation. Likewise, a maid would not be able to cultivate "Sanftmuth, Demuth und Aufopferungsfähigkeit" (*Emancipation* 82) because of her underprivileged social position. For this reason, Dohm can speak of "roh geartete Frauen der niedersten Klassen" (*Emancipation* 128). Similarly, a high-society lady will develop a completely different set of personality traits:

> Eine gewisse Sanftmuth oder Indolenz des äußeren Wesens wird sich häufig als Merkmal ihrer [der Salondame] ausgepolsterten Existenz bei ihr einstellen, und der zarte Parfum ihres Charakters und ihres Schnupftuches wird nicht verfehlen, sie in den Augen erfahrener Menschenkenner und Psychologen mit der Aureole edler Weiblichkeitr zu schmücken. (*Emancipation* 83)

Such women do not have any opportunity to develop or utilize skills or abilities that would enable them to be independent.

Likewise, Dohm dismisses Bischoff's principle of the inherent and unconquerable sensitivity of female nature. She admits that women might indeed be gentle, but they can overcome this tenderness of feelings if they want to or are forced to do so. Again, working-class women provide good examples:

> Hand aufs Herz, Herr von Bischoff, was würden Sie mit Ihrer Köchin thun, die den Aal, den Sie so gern essen, abzuschlachten sich weigerte, und sich bei Ihnen mit ihrem Zartgefühl entschuldigen wollte? Würden Sie nicht vielleicht diese Köchin gerade ihres Zartgefühls wegen entlassen, um sie durch eine Andere, frisch darauf losschlachtende zu ersetzen? (*Emancipation* 120)

Dohm contends that people, regardless of their social status, are able to suppress certain feelings and change various qualities if they are forced to adapt to particular circumstances in life. Higher-class women have the funds provided by their husbands to cultivate an exquisite life style and corresponding personality traits, but the majority of women cannot afford such an existence:

> Wenn die Köchin [...] vor ihrem zappelnden Huhn oder Fisch keiner Ohnmachtsanwandlungen sich zu unterziehen braucht, um ihre Weiblichkeit zu beweisen, wenn Sie [Prof. Bischoff] die Hebammen, Schlächterfrauen, Krankenwärterinnen u.s.w. ruhig gewähren lassen, ohne gegen sie zu polemisieren – so verdammen Sie auch die Ärztin nicht, weil sie gesunde Nerven hat, weil sie vermöge [...] gewisse Gefühlsregungen zu überwinden. (*Emancipation* 120-21)

Female physicians are able to do voluntarily what poor women are forced to do because of their social status—to suppress any gentleness that could interfere with their work. In the face of poverty and hunger, most women would do anything to save themselves and their children from death. The so-called female "Zartgefühl," as defined by Bischoff, is just a luxurious commodity on the high-society marriage market and a middle-class male fantasy. In addition, it serves as a pretext to keep women away from higher education, especially from medical schools (*Emancipation* 85).

According to Dohm, Bischoff confuses "schwache Nerven oder Zartgefühl für 'die elegante Welt' mit dem wahren Zartgefühl, das allein auf der Gesinnung beruht und nicht im Auf- und Niederzucken von einem Paar Nerven besteht" (*Emancipation* 121). The first type of "sensitivity" is a gender construct acquired by upper-class women as a result of upbringing and specific "husband-oriented education." It is a superficial quality put on mainly for show by upper-class women to display their so-called femininity. According to Dohm, this type of sensitivity manifests itself through "schleunige Gefühlseruptionen" and "Virtuosität im Ekeln" (*Emancipation* 121). However, this type of sensitivity is not only a consequence of family role models and specific upbringing; it is also a result of the empty and meaningless life that upper-class women are forced to lead. Dohm implies the performative character of class and gender, concepts that are fundamental to twentieth-century feminist criticism:

> [L]iebenswürdige Damen der Gesellschaft, angebleicht und angekränkelt von *poudre de riz* und tausend und einem Roman und versehen mit der ganzen üblichen Garderobe des Zartgefühls: Nervenzucken, Parfüm, Spitzen und Fächer u.s.w., werden meistentheils vor einem Seciertisch in Ohnmacht fallen. Diese Feinfühligkeit wird sie aber unter Umständen nicht hindern, durch raffinierte Koketterie ein treues Herz zu martern oder das Lebensglück einer ehrenwerthen Mitschwester durch niederträchtige Verleumdung zu zerstören. Seien Sie unbesorgt, meine Damen, derartige kleine Salonscherze werden den Ruf Ihrer zarten Weiblichkeit nicht compromittieren, so lange die Männer dekretieren, was weiblich und was unweiblich zu thun und zu wissen ist! (*Emancipation* 122)

Although this kind of "sensitivity" is class-specific, Bischoff argues that it is inborn and disqualifies all women from entering medical schools. By using the expression "Garderobe des Zartgefühls," Dohm emphasizes that upper- and middle-class femininity is indeed a performance. The superficial "Zartgefühl" has a demonstrative character and is, like *poudre de riz*, merely a type of make-up used by upper-class women to perform their class and gender roles. These women are not allowed to become authentic human beings due to the normative pressure imposed by their surroundings. And again, such a spectacle of "noble femininity" is class-specific and based on the prescriptive character of gender roles. Bischoff's notion of femininity is a construct of a prescriptive and not of a descriptive character. It belongs to the realm of male fantasies and not to real life. The second type of "Zartgefühl" is founded in humanity and is a non-gender-specific and a non-class-specific quality. It manifests itself as love of justice and genuine concern about the sufferings of humankind and, according to Dohm, it is also a powerful motivation behind the struggle of women to gain admission to medical schools.

According to Lange, most of the upper- and middle-class women suffer "eine geistige Not" (*Frauenbildung* 81) because they do not receive any intellectual nourishment. They are not able to live a meaningful life in which they could further their own personal development. These women struggle in vain to find a purpose in their lives: "[Da] kämpft die Tochter, die nur das Leben verschönern soll, mit dem heißen Wunsch, zu nützen" (*Frauenbildung* 84). Lange calls such an existence "Geistesmord" (*Frauenbildung* 85). In addition to intellectual emptiness many middle-class women also suffer financial hardships, especially if they cannot be married off. Female access to higher education would help to eliminate both.

Class, however, proved tenacious even in these attempts to dispute its limits. As forceful as the women's call for female physicians was, it, too, was influenced by the class component. The dominant argument aimed at introducing mainly middle-class women[126] to the medical profession as physicians in order to grant them intellectual development and financial independence. At the same time, it was directed towards both middle- and lower-class women as potential patients who would profit from the option to consult female medical doctors. It is apparent, especially in the texts by Lange and Binder, that the struggle of middle-class women for admission to higher education was highly influenced by their understanding and perception of class differences. They did not even consider the possiblility of lower-class women entering universities. The financial factor definitely played a role, since the lower classes could not afford education. But this seems to be only part of the issue because many middle-class families were also impoverished and could not afford granting their daughters education. Besides, there were fellowships founded by women's organizations available to women who wanted to pursue higher education. Therefore, the exclusion of lower-class women from demands for higher education seems to have much more to do with a middle-class perception of their intellectual inadequacy.

Lange quotes an English physician, Elizabeth Garret-Anderson, to demonstrate the benefit women from different social classes would have if they could consult a female doctor: "Wir wissen sehr wohl, daß das Bedürfnis nach weiblichen Ärzten nicht in den vornehmen, sondern in den gebildeten Kreisen und unter den Armen vorhanden ist" (*Frauenbildung* 36). While educated women would be able to enter the medical profession as physicians, the lower-class women would benefit from being able to go to a female doctor. As indicated by Garret-Anderson, upper-class women are actually excluded from the need or wish to have female medical doctors available to them. Garret-Anderson claims, and Lange seems to agree with her, that aristocratic women actually "enjoy" going to a male doctor. They are women who "nur wenig Arzenei nehmen, aber gerne viele Besprechungen mit ihrem angenehmen, heiteren Arzt haben" (Garret-Anderson qtd. in Lange, *Frauenbildung* 36). Consequently, Garret-Anderson argues, upper-class women do not support the demand for female physicians because they are satisfied with the male ones. Hence, the issue has a particular significance mainly for working-class women as potential patients and for middle-class women as both potential patients and doctors.

2.7 The Dichotomy of Reason and Emotion and Other Gender-Specific Qualities

Dohm points out that in addition to prescribed sensitivity and gentleness, Bischoff defines women as lacking cognitive abilities necessary for the pursuit of an academic career. Bischoff evokes the traditional dichotomy of reason and emotion, attributing the former to men and the latter to women. Accordingly, "Unzulänglichkeit der Denkfunktionen" and "reiches Gefühlsleben" (*Emancipation* 95)

126 See also Mazón 16; 53.

constitute typically female qualities. These two features are cited as the main obstacles on the road to higher education for women. As mentioned above, Bischoff explains the underdeveloped intellectual abilities in females as a consequence of their undersized brains. Dohm rejects this line of argument as illogical. She points out that according to most medical scientists of the time, the brain is the center for both thought and feeling. Hence, if Bischoff's brain theory were accurate, females could not have simultaneously an underdeveloped intellect and overdeveloped emotions. Further, she argues against the split of reason and emotion along gender lines and points to many women driven by reason and many men consumed by strong emotions. She concludes that all people, regardless of their biological sex, act both reasonably and emotionally. At the same time, however, she recognizes that men have an aversion to acknowledging women in the intellectual sphere: "Tief eingewurzelt ist der Widerwille der Männer, die Frau auf geistigem Gebiet anzuerkennen" (*Emancipation* 45).

Although Dohm asserts that women have the same intellectual potential as men, she recognizes that women were deliberately raised in the belief that thinking was a male domain:

> Es ist den Frauen unaufhörlich eingeschärft worden: für Euch denken die Männer, - daß sie schließlich aufgehört haben zu denken. Lange Reihen von Frauengenerationen sind unter dem Drucke der Verachtung ihrer Intelligenz aufgewachsen, und natürlich haben sie etwas gethan um diese Verachtung zu rechtfertigen. (*Emancipation* 61)

Many women have abandoned their need for intellectual development, choosing instead to perform their prescribed gender role. For most of them, however, it was not a matter of choice but an imposed social position due to the patriarchal structure of Western society and its gender politics.

Dohm points out that the schools for middle-class girls, institutions that should be responsible for the intellectual development of their pupils, only perpetuate this situation: "Wie systematisch das Denkvermögen in den Mädchenschulen untergraben wird" (*Emancipation* 34). Instead of granting young women appropriate intellectual development, they prepare them for the "mindless" life of the typical bourgeois wife. As discussed earlier, because the idea of a well-educated and intellectually developed woman did not appeal to the average male taste, the female pursuit of knowledge was not only discouraged but, more importantly, was made almost impossible.

Lange also objects to this aspect of gender politics: "Die irren sicher, die da meinen, Bildung thue für den Mann alles, für die Frau nichts" (Lange 105). Although she agrees with the statement: "[D]as Beste an der Frau sei etwas ganz anderes als das Wissen" (*Frauenbildung* 104), she also maintains that education for middle-class women is as important as it is for men. In addition, she argues that the overriding public fear of educated women is relatively new and typical especially for the nineteenth century: "Die Furcht vor einer gründlichen Frauenbildung ist selbst in Deutschland spezifisch modern; das Mittelalter kannte sie nicht. Erst unsere Zeit ist die Schöpferin des 'Blaustrumpfes'" (*Frauenbildung* 105). She further contends that it is precisely the male attempt to suppress female intellectual development that produces the feared result in the form of degenerate, melancholic, and sickly individuals. In her book, Lange attests to a woman's longing for serious intellectual and professional work: "[D]ie Sehnsucht nach ernsthafter Geistes- und Berufsarbeit" (*Frauenbildung* 85). Morgenstern perceives a specific female drive to which she refers as "ein wissenschaftlicher, höherer Trieb" (6) and as "innerste geistige Neigung, ein seelisches Dürsten" (20). According to her, this drive is the main cause of women's demands for higher education. Such a claim negates the typically male perception of the time, which reduces women to the physical dimension and denies them access to the intellectual realm. It also reinforces the idea that women, like men, are able to transcend their physicality and are capable of more than just "sexuelle[s] Gefühlsleben" (Weber 41).

According to Bischoff, a whole subset of male and female qualities complements the gender-specific assignment of reason and emotion. As a result of the gender-specific separation of characteristics, each sex is constructed as the exact opposite of the other. According to this gender model, women and men do not have any common personality traits nor do they share any qualities. Dohm criticizes such a gender paradigm as being completely inadequate and simplistic: "[G]leich wie in jener mythologischen Dichtung Sonne und Mond sich ewig suchen und ewig fliehen, so kommen Mann und Weib in ihrem Seelenleben nie zusammen! Wo der Eine aufhört, ideal zu sein, fängt der Andere erst an" (*Emancipation* 135). In this division, characteristics condemning an individual to the private sphere are attributed only to women. By the same token, personality traits predisposing a person to an adventurous or intellectual life outside the house are ascribed to men. Dohm points out that Bischoff imprints the so-called "male characteristics" with a positive connotation and does the opposite with "female qualities." A quality, by virtue of being ascribed to one of the sexes, usually evokes rather positive associations if it is ascribed to men and carries negative overtones if it is attributed to women.[127] Correspondingly, even objectively negative characteristics such as "Rohheit" and "Gefühllosigkeit" (Dohm, *Emancipation* 124) seem to lose their negative meaning if they are exhibited by men. In women they are completely unacceptable. Similarly, "Sinnlichkeit" in women is a negative trait, while in men it is a positive one (Dohm, *Emancipation* 81). Lange also indicates that the notion of femininity carries a whole set of negative, socially constructed associations that diminish female humanity: "Weiblichkeit! Schönes, gemißhandeltes Wort! Was liegt nicht alles darin: Liebe, Vertrauen, Idealismus,

127 See also Schmersahl 328-29.

Opfermut und Seelengröße! Und was möchte man damit verbinden? Zimperlichkeit und Unnatur" (*Frauenbildung* 113).

Dohm further points out that Bischoff starts with the assumption that women are not able to study medicine and then tries to find all the qualities that make such a pursuit impossible. Subsequently, he attributes such characteristics to all women. According to Dohm, Bischoff follows this logic and "begnügt sich mit der Annahme hypothetischer Eigenschaften, die für seine Vorurtheile passen" (*Emancipation* 79). His list of "typical" female and male characteristics is based on the traditional view of gender distinctiveness:

> Der Mann ist muthig, kühn, heftig, trotzig, rauh, verschlossen; das Weib furchtsam, nachgiebig, sanft, zärtlich, gutmüthig, geschwätzig, verschmitzt. Der Mann besitzt mehr Festigkeit, das Weib ist wandelbar und inconsequent. Der Mann handelt nach Überzeugungen, das Weib nach Gefühlen; die Vernunft beherrscht bei jenem das Gefühl, bei diesem umgekehrt das Gefühl die Vernunft. [...] Das Weib ist schamhafter und die Regungen des groben Genusses der Sinnlichkeit sind bei ihm in der Regel geringer, als bei dem Manne. Der Mann ist das Schaffende, das Weib das erhaltende Prinzip der menschlichen Gesellschaft. (Bischoff 19-20; qtd. in Dohm, *Emancipation* 78-79)

By challenging Bischoff's notion of male and female characteristics, Dohm attempts to undermine the traditional understanding of gender and negotiate new roles for women: "Tausende von Frauen sind klüger, heftiger, muthiger als Tausende von Männern, und Tausende von Männern sind sanfter, aufopferungsfähiger, gutmüthiger als Tausende von Frauen" (*Emancipation* 85). She emphasizes that these traits are not gender-specific, but are shared by all human beings. Women are able to enrich society through intellectual and creative achievements on the basis of their skills and abilities to the same degree as men. The only difference is that women have been prevented from utilizing their talents: "Wir [Frauen] besitzen alle Seelenschätze der Welt; sie haben nur einen Fehler: sie nützen uns nichts" (*Emancipation* 66). Dohm refers to an old tale in which fairies gave every conceivable magnificent personality and character traits to a newborn prince. Unfortunately, the family forgot to invite one fairy who decided to take revenge for this insult by making all the gifts useless and unprofitable. Dohm reads this story as an allegory of the female existence: women are intellectually capable of pursuing higher education but this quality seems to be useless because they are not permitted to obtain academic degrees.

3 The Female Body and Regulatory Practices in the Public and Private Space

> *Women and men are spatially segregated in ways that reduce women's access to knowledge and thereby reinforce women's lower status relative to men's. "Gendered spaces" separate women from knowledge used by men to produce and reproduce power and privilege.*
>
> Daphne Spain[128]

3.1 Introduction: Intersections of Space, Gender, and Class

In an article published in *Die Frauenbewegung* in December 1897, Marie Raschke relates the following incident:

> Ein ehrbares, unbescholtenes Mädchen geht an einem Sommerabend in Berlin nach der Brunnenstraße, um ihren Bräutigam, der in den Elektrizitätswerken angestellt ist, abzuholen. Sie wird von einem rohen Gesellen angeredet, dessen sie sich mit den Worten erwehrt: "Belästigen Sie mich nicht!" Bald darauf kehrt der Mann mit einem Polizeibeamten wieder, der sie anredet: "Fräulein, Sie sollen diesen Herrn hier angekobert haben; er verlangt Ihre Feststellung; Sie müssen mit zur Wache." [...] Das Mädchen wird darauf die Nacht über auf der Polizei behalten, am folgenden Morgen im grünen Wagen nach dem Polizeipräsidium gefahren, ärztlicher Untersuchung unterworfen und erst nachmittags um 2 Uhr [...] auf freien Fuß gesetzt. ("Die weibliche Ehre" 250)

The above passage exemplifies the main themes of this chapter. It demonstrates that a single woman's presence in the public space was suspect and indicates that a virtuous middle-class woman belonged primarily in the private realm. It also reveals certain regulatory practices in the public space over which men had absolute control. Additionally, the passage suggests that this young woman was reduced to a sexualized body. First she was turned into an object of male sexual desire by the harasser and later she was arrested as a potential prostitute by a police officer. The gynecological exam performed on the girl suspected of prostitution heightens awareness of the need for female medical doctors.

This particular incident is important not only because it addresses some of the main themes of this book, but also because the described situation and the women's struggle for admission to universities and medical schools have much in

128 Spain 3.

common: both are embedded in a broader nexus of space and gender. As Linda McDowell and Joanne P. Sharp note:

> The dualism of home/workplace, the public sphere and the private arena, is mapped onto and constructs a gendered difference between male and female that has taken a particular special form in western nations since the industrial revolution. Although it has long been recognized that this division is an imperfect one, as millions of women have worked for wages of some sort outside and inside their homes, its significance rests in its normative function. Women who are "out of place" – in the streets, in the workplace, in public – are seen in some senses as unnatural or unsexed. (263)

As indicated by McDowell and Sharp, the construction of a gendered difference between men and women rests upon a specific division of space. However, I argue that in addition to gender differences being supported by the duality of the public and private realm, the space itself is gendered. Furthermore, I intend to demonstrate that the relationship between space and gender is much more complex than the above passage suggests. Women who are "out of place" are not only perceived as "unnatural or unsexed." They can also be objectified in a very sexual way, as is the girl in Raschke's article, depending on their location within the public realm. Lynne Walker, for instance, distinguishes between the respectable feminine place in the private realm and a sexually charged presence outside: "At mid-century, middle-class woman's place in the home distinguished respectable femininity in opposition to the prostitute, the fallen woman of the streets" (65).

Due to the intersections of social status and gender discussed in Chapter Two, the gender/space nexus is further complicated by the class factor.[129] Since it was relatively easy for a viewer to immediately establish a person's social status based on her appearance, the female body acquired a particular meaning based on its location and on the external class markers (for example, clothing, jewelry or lack thereof, hair style). Adding the space and class factors to the discussion of gender differences, we are actually presented with many varieties of the female gender.

The relationship between space and gender is reciprocal. The division between the public and private realm is discursively translated into the division between men and women. By the same token space is gendered.[130] At the end of

---

129 Pollock also makes the connection between space, class, and gender. She writes: "The [...] territories of the bourgeois city were [...] not only gendered on a male/female polarity. They became the sites for the negotiation of gendered class identities and class gender positions. The spaces of modernity are where class and gender interface in critical ways, in that they are the spaces of sexual exchange" (70).

130 See also Pollock's discussion of gendered spaces in the context of late nineteenth-century art 56; 66-70. She writes: "[T]he mapping of the separation of the spheres for women and men

the nineteenth century, certain places such as streets, universities, libraries, offices, etc., were perceived as exclusively male domains in which men enjoyed numerous privileges. In contrast, women were restricted mainly to the private realm. Walker notes a similar situation in the British context in which "the identity of Victorian women was closely bound up in the home and their removal from public life" (65). Walker further claims that the separation of the male and female spheres "was deeply drawn between the public (masculine) world of remuneration, work and recognition and the private (feminine) domestic realm of home and family responsibilities" (65).

Although certain women were "allowed" to enter the male realm, such a transgression was usually justified only in terms of male pleasure or profit and was perceived as socially degrading because primarily two types of lower-class women came into the male-dominated public space: the working woman and the prostitute. As discussed in the previous chapter, working-class men and women were believed to exhibit fewer gender differences than persons of the upper classes. Hence, the working-class woman was de-feminized and consequently de-sexualized in the eyes of upper- and middle-class men.[131] At the same time, the prostitute was reduced to a sexual object available to any man. In other words, a woman's presence in places identified with the male realm had a direct impact on how her womanhood was perceived. When measured against these principles, a middle-class woman's entrance into the public space carried a number of potentially negative consequences. Such a woman would surrender the respectable position she enjoyed in the private realm due to her social status as a wife and/or mother. Upon entering the public space reserved for men and to which only lower-class women were admitted, the body of a middle-class woman would be publicly degraded, de-feminized, or sexually charged.[132] It is not surprising that this discursively constructed reciprocal relation between femininity and the public space also negatively affected the popular perception of women demanding admission to universities.

---

on to the division of public and private was powerfully operative in the construction of a specifically bourgeois way of life" (68) and "The public and private division functioned on many levels. As a metaphorical map in ideology, it structured the very meaning of the terms masculine and feminine within its mythic boundaries. In practice as the ideology of domesticity became hegemonic, it regulated women's and men's behaviour in the respective public and private spaces. Presence in either of the domains determined one's social identity [...]" (69).

131 See also Pollock 68-69.

132 Pollock makes a similar observation in relation to various public places. She writes: "To enter such spaces as the masked ball or the café-concert constituted a serious threat to a bourgeois woman's reputation and therefore her femininity. The guarded respectability of the lady could be soiled by mere visual contact for seeing what was bound up with knowing. This other world of encounter between bourgeois men and women of another class was a no-go area for bourgeois women" (78). See also Pollock 78-79.

3.2 One Female Sex and Multiple Gender Types[133]

Medical discourses in conjunction with responses by female authors produced a number of gender variations with regard to women in general. Seemanthini Niranjana suggests, in a different context, a diversity of discourses and practices that produced gendered identities: "[T]he category of gender implied not merely sexual or biological differences between the male and female, but also the social recreation or construction of gendered identities. These were seen as produced by a range of socio-cultural and material practices, institutional-ideological discourses, and the practices of daily life" (14). Such a multiplicity, in turn, blurs a clear-cut distinction between men and women. During the second half of the nineteenth century, medical discourses attempted to create standards of sexual behaviors and classify human beings according to the degree to which they adhered to the prescribed sexual norms.[134] These discourses and practices not only produced numerous gendered identities, but also multiplied the biological categories by adding the hermaphrodite to the standard male and female sex.[135]

Based on the reciprocal triangle of space, gender, and class, these discourses created five female gender types: the working-class woman, the maid, the upper- and middle-class woman, the prostitute, and the female student. The multiplicity of female gender models is based on the specific sexual, reproductive, and biological functions that are mapped onto the female body in five different ways. By the end of the nineteenth century the first four types constituted gender patterns already well established in Austria and Germany, but the female student emerged as a new and suspect phenomenon.[136]

---

133 Anne Fausto-Sterling argues in her book *Sexing the Body. Gender Politics and the Construction of Sexuality* that throughout history, construction of multiple genders corresponded to the two sexes. For example, in the eighteenth century there were two sexes and three genders (women, heterosexual men, and homosexual men); in the course of the nineteenth century, the discourses split women into two genders: heterosexual and homosexual; and in the late nineteenth century, scientists classified numerous sexes and genders. Finally, contemporary science distinguishes six genders: heterosexual men and women, gay men and lesbians, and bisexual men and women (Fausto-Sterling 11). The title of this subchapter, however, refers to five female types present in the discussion about female admission to medical schools.

134 See also Thorson 6-7; Schmersahl 39-113. Schmersahl argues that by labeling particular behaviors as normal or abnormal, the medical discourse had a normative function; it could "im Namen der Wissenschaft und der Gesundheit von der gängigen Meinung abweichende Einstellungen oder Lebensweisen [...] pathologisieren" (63). Consequently, medicine became a means to reinforce socially accepted behaviors: "Die medizinische Konstruktion, Beschreibung und Kategorisierung sexueller 'Perversionen' diente der Naturalisierung und Durchsetzung sozialer, und zwar vor allem geschlechtsspezifischer Verhaltensnormen" (Schmersahl 113).

135 For a discussion of the "third sex," the hermaphrodite, see Thorson 43-98.

136 Weiershausen analyzes literary representations of the female student. In this context she writes: "In der Neuheit der wissenschaftlich gebildeten Frau liegt eine besondere discursive

A working-class woman, as part of the industrial workforce (for example, mine or factory worker), inhabited both the private and the public realm. Due to late-nineteenth-century economic conditions, she was forced to undertake physical work and consequently enter the public space.[137] By virtue of her social status, she was believed to exhibit certain masculine features and to be less feminine than an upper-class woman.[138] Referring to working women, McDowell and Sharp point out that "[t]he early anxieties of the English factory inspectors that work would unfit young women for marriage was [sic] paralleled by Engels' anxiety that women's participation in the work force [...] created a 'world turned upside down'"(263). According to the German texts I discuss, the physical work itself did not diminish female reproductive functions. However, the working-class women were not perceived as objects of desire by middle-class men. In addition to this lack of desirability, the lack of educational demands by or on behalf of working-class women made them invisible in texts written by opponents of women's medical education. Consequently, this female type is characterized by an absence within the male discourses on education and sexuality.

One exception to this stereotype of the undesirable working-class woman was the stereotypical maid ("Dienstmädchen") whose body was highly sexualized and defined in terms of male pleasure. Although she shared this sexually charged perception with a prostitute, her desirability was based on her connection to the private space of the family. Unlike the body of a prostitute, her body was not "contaminated" by a presence on the street, in both a literal and metaphorical sense. Ichenhaeuser refers to an essay by a Professor Platter,[139] "Der Krieg gegen die Mütter," in which he emphasizes the extraordinary appeal of a maid due to her presence in the private realm:

> In welcher Klasse von weiblichen Wesen giebt es mehr frische, dralle, kräftige und lebenslustige Figuren als unter den *Dienstmädchen, die nichts als häusliche Arbeit verrichten?* [...] [S]ie haben *eine dem weiblichen Körper angemessene Beschäftigungs- und Le-*

Sprengkraft: Einerseits provoziert die Akademikerin Einordnungsversuche, andererseits verursacht sie den Figuren aus ihrem sozialen Umfeld Schwierigkeiten der Zuordnung" (226). See also Weiershausen 266-269.

137 I use the term "public" space to refer to any space outside the house. Although a mine or a factory is not "public" space per se because it is not freely accessible to anyone, working women had to leave the private realm to enter the work place. On the other hand, however, mines and factories are "public" spaces because in them masses of people come together.

138 See also Pollock 68. In his well-known study of fascism, Klaus Theweleit demonstrated that the perception of working-class women as being inherently different from middle-class women became even more extreme during WW I. However, it was the sexuality of these women that received monstrous dimensions. Working-class women were often equated with "whores," "monsters," "beasts" by German soldiers (1: 65-68). They were also seen as "shameless" and "threatening"(1: 68). See also Theweleit 1: 138-157.

139 His first name is unknown.

bensweise. Sie sind denn bei Heirathskandidaten des Arbeiter- und kleineren Mittelstandes die gesuchteste Ware, sie gehen ab wie frische Semmeln. (qtd. in Ichenhaeuser, *Ausnahmestellung* 11; emphasis added)

Platter presents only a one-sided male perspective on the gender status of the maid. He objectifies her, which is evident in his use of commercial language. He refers to maids as "die gesuchteste Ware" and compares them to fresh bread rolls. In so doing Platter de-humanizes these women and emphasizes their status as a sexual commodity. Similarly, his use of adjectives suggests a sexually charged perception. As highlighted in this passage, the maid's sexual appeal springs from her inclusion and presence in the private space. Ichenhaeuser makes the reasons for a male interest in maids very clear: "Jawohl, sie gehen wie frische Semmeln ab, aber nicht zum heiraten, sondern zum amüsieren" (*Ausnahmestellung* 12).

Unlike the working-class woman, a woman from the upper and middle class was perceived as the essence of femininity. She remained exclusively in the private realm, satisfied her purpose in life by serving her husband and by giving birth to his children.[140] She was the passive body without a voice per se. Although she was reduced to a sexualized body,[141] the reproductive function, unlike that of the prostitute, gave her existence an additional meaning because she gave birth to "honorable" offspring. It is evident that her most important feature was her ability to reproduce. However, it is noteworthy that at the end of the nineteenth century many critical writings followed Marx and Engels by comparing middle-class women to prostitutes since an upper- and middle-class marriage involved both financial and sexual transactions. The middle-class woman and her body were the actual targets of the public debate about the admission of women to universities and medical schools.

While the middle-class woman's body was classified in terms of reproduction, the prostitute's body was defined in terms of pleasure. The middle-class woman gave birth to "honorable" citizens, and thus she participated in the

140 See also Schmersahl 71-72. Schmersahl makes the connection between "scientific" views of female sexuality and women's exclusion from the public realm: "Die in der Jahrhunderthälfte vorherrschende Bestimmung von weiblicher Sexualität, nämlich kaum existent und passiv zu sein, in Verbindung mit dem angeblichen Geschlechtscharakteristikum mangelnder Selbstbeherrschung, führte im Rahmen der Vorstellungen über die kulturhistorische Funktion von Sexualität dazu, den Frauen – nunmehr naturwissenschaftlich legitimiert – ihre Eignung für jegliche Teilnahme an der bürgerlichen Öffentlichkeit abzusprechen" (71).

141 By "a sexualized body," I mean that a middle-class woman was perceived as such by her husband but was not supposed to have sexual desires of her own. Schmersahl points out that Richard von Krafft-Ebing and Cesare Lombroso propagated such a view of female sexuality: "Ist es [das Weib] geistig normal entwickelt und wohlerzogen, so ist sein sinnliches Verlangen ein geringes. Wäre dem nicht so, so müsste die ganze Welt ein Bordell und Ehe und Familie undenkbar sein" (qtd. in Schmersahl 72).

reproduction of the nation.[142] The prostitute, however, did not participate in the reproduction of the nation in this fashion, because her body was "contaminated" by her profession and by her perpetual presence in the public realm. In his critical analysis of the social meaning of prostitution, Thomas Laqueur argues that in the nineteenth century prostitutes were believed to be infertile:

> Prostitutes were generally regarded as an unproductive commodity. Because they were public women; because their reproductive organs bore such heavy traffic; because in them the semen of so many different men was mixed, pell-mell, together; because the ovaries of prostitutes, through overstimulation, were seldom without morbid lesions; because their Fallopian tubes were closed by excessive intercourse; or, most tellingly, because they did not feel affection for the men with whom they had sex, they were thought to be barren, or in any case unlikely to have children. (230)

In her book *Sklavenketten der Frauen* (1893), Rosa Stolle calls attention to the polarization between the public realm of pleasure embodied by the prostitute and the private realm of reproduction personified by the bourgeois wife: "Die Aerzte sagen zu einem Ehemann: 'Ihre Frau muß geschont werden, ohne weiblichen Umgang können Sie aber nicht leben, das ist ungesund für Sie, Sie finden solche Frauenzimmer ja auch zu Dutzenden'"(56). Stolle also points out that such reasoning validates the existence of prostitution as a necessary part of the public realm, although at the same time society condemns the institutionalized sexual exchange: "[J]eder verachtet eine öffentliche Dirne, und doch werden die Prostituierten dem Staate einverleibt wie Kirche und Schule, Gericht und Militär" (50). Although the prostitute as a gender type was the subject of numerous medical, sociological, and psychological studies that focused on female sexuality and criminal behavior, she did not enter the discourses on the female body and sexuality in the context of women's education.

As a result of the public discussion of women's academic education a new gender type emerged: the female student.[143] The female student, to whom opponents of women's education also referred as "Mannweib," was discursively constructed as a highly unfeminine and completely de-sexualized being. In some

142 Schmersahl writes: "Die Familie gewinnt ihren politischen Rang als Stütze staatlicher Gewalt, die im 'pater familias' ihren Bürgen findet, in ihrer Aufgabe als Sozialisierungsinstanz für den künftigen Untertan und die Festschreibung der Geschlechterrollen. Die Frau als Gattin, Hausfrau und erziehende Mutter wurde damit zur unerläßlichen Bedingung für die Existenz des Staates" (72). She also quotes Krafft-Ebing on the issue: "Mag auch die Natur bloss Fortpflanzung fordern, so kann ein Gemeinwesen (Familie oder Staat) nicht bestehen ohne Garantie, dass das Erzeugte physisch, moralisch und intellectuell gedeihe" (Schmersahl 72).

143 See also Weiershausen 226; 266-269.

writings, animal features such as "Rabenstimme" (Dohm, *Emancipation* 174) were imposed on the female student. Such women were described as possessing masculine characteristics and as unable to fulfill their reproductive functions and/or duties.[144] Their transgression was twofold. Female students not only entered the public space of the university that had been reserved for men, but they also transgressed the boundaries of the previously exclusive gendered knowledge. It is obvious that measured against the prevailing middle-class standards of femininity and masculinity, these women did not fit into either of the two categories. Therefore, it is not surprising to see them situated in a kind of "gender no-man's land."[145]

Dohm points out that women who managed to gain admission to universities must have possessed exceptional qualities such as "außergewöhnliche Begabung," "energischen und ungewöhnlich edlen Character," "starke[...] Energie," and "Originalität des Denkens" (*Emancipation* 47-49). Dohm further refers to women who studied at the university in Zurich as "heldenmüthige Mädchen von feuriger Initiative" (*Emancipation* 52). She makes it very apparent that female students had to exhibit personality traits conventionally perceived as male in order to be able to pursue an academic education. At a time when scientists and medical doctors made desperate attempts to hold onto clear-cut gender distinctions driven by male supremacy, such manifestations of female identity threatened to destabilize their gender ideology. Since a co-existence of both the male-oriented gender ideology and social acceptance of women publicly displaying "male qualities" was not possible, one of these principles had to be disqualified. The women's struggle for admission to medical schools and universities boils down to a clash of the two principles in which male scientists try to reinforce the notion of pathological roots of such manifestations of female identity,[146] and progressive activists and writers strive to change the gender ideology of the time.[147] In his influential book, *Making Sex. Body and Gender from the Greeks to Freud*, Laqueur suggests that

144 See also Weiershausen 46-47.

145 While analyzing Lou Andreas-Salomé's novel *Fenitschka*, Weiershausen points out that the protagonist, a female student, irritates the main male character, Max Werner, "weil er sie hinsichtlich ihrer sexuellen Disposition nicht einordnen kann. Die gängigen Verhaltensregeln, die eine Einordnung zulassen würden, finden auf diese Frau keine Anwendung mehr" (132). Weiershausen also argues that in this novel "die gesellschaftlich vorgegebenen Bilder von Weiblichkeit [...] am konkreten Beispiel der Studentin scheitern. Die Begrenztheit dieser Bilder offenbart, daß es sich lediglich um Konstruktionen handelt, die nicht mit der Wirklichkeit übereinstimmen" (133).

146 Schmersahl argues throughout her book that in the nineteenth-century medical discourse, women who did not adhere to socially acceptable gender roles were branded as deviant. She writes, for example: "Jede Grenzüberschreitung dieser als 'Biologie' definierten 'weiblichen Natur' führte ihrer [der Mediziner] Meinung nach zu 'Krankheit' oder 'Entartung. ' Damit konnte jede Form des Aufbegehrens von Frauen pathologisiert und auf diese Weise ihres gesellschaftspolitischen Inhalts beraubt werden" (344).

147 See also Thorson 8. Schmersahl characterizes this struggle in a similar way: "In dieser von vielen Zeitgenossenn als kriesenhaft empfundenen Zeit verdichtete sich auch der medizi-

[t]he dominant [...] view since the eighteenth century has been that there are two stable, incommensurable, opposite sexes and the political, economic, and cultural lives of men and women, their gender roles, are somehow based on these "facts." Biology—the stable, ahistorical, sexed body—is understood to be the epistemic foundation for prescriptive claims about the social order. (6)

Precisely this dominant view of the biologically based woman's status in society was being challenged by the feminists at the end of the nineteenth century.

In Chapters One and Two, I highlighted numerous inconsistencies in the arguments of opponents of women's medical education with regard to the abilities and characteristics of women who would potentially pursue an academic education. These inconsistencies attest to the fact that the female student is a newly emerging gender type materializing through the practices and discourses of the time. An educated middle-class woman freely transgressing the public space and the boundaries of gendered knowledge was definitely a new phenomenon, and one with which society at large did not feel comfortable. She "committed" this transgression not to please or satisfy men, but in order to gain the means for financial independence while developing her own intellectual potential. Since only the prostitute and the working-class woman were tolerated by men in the public space, and because the middle-class woman was bound to the private realm,[148] the appearance of female students in the public space of the university created a particular gender confusion that did not exist before. Therefore, labeling female students in terms of gender and sexuality became rather problematic. This new gender type seemed to inherit different qualities from the other female types. On the one hand, the female student was associated with the noble femininity by virtue of belonging to the middle class. On the other hand, however, her presence in the public space was linked to low social class and to morally degrading behavior. Through their presence in the public realm among men, female students acquired the status of sexual objects and were compared to prostitutes; hence they were often suspected of loose sexual behavior. At the same time, however, these women were deemed not desirable to men because their intellect and level of knowledge corresponding to

---

nische Diskurs zur Geschlechterordnung [...]: Ärzte sahen sich massiv durch die Emanzipationsbestrebungen von Frauen bedroht. Deswegen funktionalisierten sie ihr 'Wissen' über das 'Wesen' der Frau gegen eine befürchtete Um- bzw. Neustrukturierung der Geschlechterverhältnisse" (302).

148 Pollock writes: "[...] a woman going out to dine at a restaurant even with her husband present was scandalous whereas a man dining out with a mistress, even in the view of his friends, was granted a fictive invisibility" (69). [Pollock's footnote in this passage refers to Richard Sennett's *The Fall of the Public Man,* Cambridge, Cambridge University Press, 1977, 23]. From the context, it is clear that the woman who does not dare to go dining with her husband belongs to the middle-class. The mistress is most probably a member of a lower social class.

academic requirements were believed to have developed at the cost of their sexuality.

The confusion as to the sexuality and consequently the womanliness of female students, particularly medical students, is further manifested through metaphorical/symbolic female types that emerge in the discourse regarding the admission of women to the universities. The most prominent types are the "Mannweib," the Vestal Virgin, the hetaera, the "Bluestocking," and the castrating woman. Such a formal typology is certainly not intended by medical doctors opposing female education and does not constitute any firm model of gender classification. Nevertheless, these five discursive variations of the female student type do occur in the texts discussing the potential entrance of women to the academic field and reflect the underlying male anxiety about shifting gender roles. Unlike the five women types discussed earlier (the working-class woman, the maid, the upper- and middle-class woman, the prostitute, and the female student), the symbolic types (the "Mannweib," the Vestal Virgin, the hetaera, the "Bluestocking," and the castrating woman) are, for the most part, not real and therefore they illustrate male anxieties regarding changing gender roles to a much higher degree than the former ones.

The female student was very often referred to as "Mannweib." As I have noted before, women attempting to study at the university were believed to be less feminine than other women because such a pursuit did not correspond with what were believed to be typically feminine qualities. Hence, the female student was perceived as "eine weibliche Form des Mannes, keine Frau mehr" (H. Fehling qtd. in Rohner 67).[149] Johannes Scherr referred to academically educated and independent women as "widerwärtige Zwitterwesen, die alles Gute des eigenen Geschlechts eingebüßt haben und alles Schlechte des männlichen angenommen haben" (Scherr qtd. in Troll-Borostyáni, "Etwas über Weiblichkeit" 812). One could add countless other examples. The underlying anxiety for men here seems to have been the potential loss of feminine appeal, attraction, and reproduction.

The confusion regarding the womanliness of the discursively constructed female student manifested itself in inconsistencies in defining her sexuality. In some texts the female student was seen as unable to reproduce or unappealing sexually to any man ("Mannweib" type). Other texts, however, portrayed her as a sexual object and target of advances and assaults by male students (and implicitly even professors). In many cases, she was believed to be sexually available to men due to her alleged low moral standards. In an extremely misogynistic article, Fritz Wittels equates the female student with the prostitute: "Man kann von den Studenten, die starke Ausdrücke lieben, oftmals hören, die weiblichen Kollegen kämen ihnen vor wie Prostituierte" (Avicenna 14-15).[150] In this case a transgression of the boundaries of knowledge was simultaneously a transgression of moral standards (hetaera type). But a number of authors also pointed out that some

149 His first name is unknown.

150 Tichy provides the real name (Fritz Wittels) of the author writing under the pseudonym "Avicenna" ("Die geschlechtliche Un-Ordnung" 40).

women would not marry, not because of their lack of femininity, but because there were more women than men in the population. In the case of these women, an academic education would be a kind of necessary substitute for marriage and would not imply "immoral behavior" ("Vestal Virgin" type).

Unlike the "Mannweib," the "Vestal Virgin" is not referred to as such in the literature debating the issue of higher education of women,[151] but I would like to propose that the female student is on many occasions discursively paralleled with the Roman priestess by virtue of similar qualities independently attributed to both. The most obvious similarity between the Roman priestess of antiquity and the female student of the nineteenth century (as she was constructed in many antagonistic texts) is the renunciation of sexual activities upon entering the transcendental realm of spirituality or knowledge. The female student had to demonstrate (perform) sexual restraint and unavailability in order to maintain a respectable position in society, in general, and at the university, in particular. Consequently, the female student, like the Vestal Virgin, had to transcend her bodily boundaries to enter the realm of knowledge and had to devote a considerable amount of time to this pursuit. The worship of Vesta is thus transformed into the devotion to science. According to the *Encyclopaedia Britannica*, Vestal Virgins could marry after they had completed their religious service. However, "few did, as it was considered unlucky" ("Vestal Virgin." *Encyclopaedia Britannica*, CD-ROM). The Roman fear of bad luck upon marrying a former Vestal Virgin is again paralleled by the notion that women who successfully graduate from a university are likely to be infertile or to deteriorate physically after giving birth. Ichenhaeuser points out that Professor Platter (against whom she argues in her text *Die Ausnahmestellung Deutschlands in Sachen des Frauenstudiums*) tries to convince his audience of multiple negative consequences following woman's entrance into the realm of higher education by extensively quoting his American colleague (not identified by name in the text) who argued that women educated at the university "schon vor der Hochzeit dermassen physisch erschöpft seien, dass sie nach der Geburt eines oder zweier Kinder zu Ruinen würden" (qtd. in Ichenhaeuser, *Ausnahmestellung* 9). Additionally, they would become "Statt einer Hülfe [..] ihrem Manne eine Bürde" (qtd. in Ichenhaeuser, *Ausnahmestellung* 8). Moreover, like Vestal Virgins, female students enjoyed a certain amount of emancipation.

151 The only exception I found is a passage from a text by A. Sieghart, *Die Frage der Frauenemanzipation. Von der höheren Weltordnung aus und in Liebe und Frauenwürde im Alterthum, Ritterthum und der Gegenwart behandelt. Gewidmet den Frauen Wiens* (qtd. in Tichy, "Die geschlechtliche Un-Ordnung" 38). The passage reads as follows: "Wenn heroische oder geistige Größe ungewöhnlich bei den Männern ist, um wie mehr erscheint sie bei den Frauen als Ausnahme; doch die Frauen, die sie besitzen, müssen 'Vestalinen' ihrer Größe bleiben, denn nicht irdische Liebe darf sie profanieren. [...] Sie wandeln auf den Bahnen der Männergröße, diese starken Frauenseelen; denn sie eignen sich nicht und können sich auch nie ins Familienleben einzwängen."

The third type corresponding to the imagined negative qualities of the female student is the hetaera, a figure who combines both education and sexual availability. As noted in the *Encyclopaedia Britannica*, the hetaera was a woman belonging to "a class of professional independent courtesans of ancient Greece who, besides developing physical beauty, cultivated their minds and talents to a degree far beyond that granted to the average Attic woman. [...], their freedom was greater than that of the married woman, who was bound to seclusion" ("Hetaera." *Encyclopaedia Britannica*, CD-ROM). Despite a potentially negative connotation, however, this type could have been appealing to some women who wanted to liberate themselves from being reduced entirely to the objects of male pleasure in order to gain freedom to enter the public realm and achieve a certain amount of autonomy and independence. Marianne Hainisch, for instance, perceives "Hetärenthum" to be "trotz seiner physischen Seite, ein Flüchten vom bloßen Geschlechtswesen zur geistig entwickelten Frau" (*Seherinnen* 8). For Franziska zu Reventlow, otherwise not engaged in the struggle for the admission of women to universities, but openly advocating female emancipation from the constraints of bourgeois sexual morality, the hetaera is a symbol of women's sexual liberation (Krause 88). However, as Krause suggests, "Dieses Verständnis des Hetärismus, [deutet] [...] allerdings den Anspruch auf intellektuelles Leben zumindest an [...]" (88).

The term "Bluestocking" was first used in England. Beatrix Schmaußer traces its origins to the mid-eighteenth century as follows. When the word was introduced in the intellectual salons of London, it had a positive meaning; it designated a shift from pointless gossiping to meaningful conversations about art, philosophy, science, and literature (Schmaußer 144). According to *Encyclopaedia Britannica*, these intellectual discussions were initiated by several upper-class women who "invited members of the aristocracy with literary interests" to these casual gatherings. *Encyclopaedia Britannica* provides the following explanation of the term's origins:

> The term probably originated when one of the ladies, Mrs. Vesey, invited the learned Benjamin Stillingfleet to one of her parties; he declined because he lacked appropriate dress, whereupon she told him to come "in his blue stockings"–the ordinary worsted stockings he was wearing at the time. He did so, and Bluestocking [...] society became a nickname for the group. This anecdote was later recounted by Madame d'Arblay (the diarist and novelist better known as Fanny Burney), one of the most famous of the Bluestockings. ("Bluestocking." *Encyclopaedia Britannica*, CD-ROM)

Under the influence of the French Revolution, Schmaußer continues, a number of "Bluestocking-Salons" were created in which important social issues such as women's inequality were discussed. The term acquired its negative meaning after the publication of Mary Wollstonecraft's *The Rights of Woman* in 1792, in which she publicized the progressive ideas developed in "Bluestocking-Salons." Thereafter, the word "Bluestocking" was used as a derogatory epithet for women who did not want to lead a conventional female existence (Schmaußer 144-45). The noun "Blaustrumpf" and the adjective "blaustrümpfig" were widely used during the debate about the admission of women to the medical profession in Austria and Germany to designate the women's lack of physical attraction, an "overdeveloped" intellect, and the demands of gender equality, in other words everything that a female student seemed to represent. Again, the popular and (pseudo) scientific literature of the time abounds with different variations of this designation. Dohm, for instance, points out that "[e]in geistreicher Feuilletonist der Nationalzeitung nennt [...] Sappho 'ein älteres blaustrümpfiges Frauenzimmer' [...]" (*Emancipation* 64-65). Anna Beruna shows that women were labeled "Blaustrümpfe" for any transgression into the realm that had been designated as the male sphere. Even a very talented woman could not pursue higher education: "Da tönt ihr [...] plötzlich und unvermittelt ein gebieterisches 'Halt' entgegen: 'nicht weiter, sonst wirst du ein Blaustrumpf!'" (Beruna 15). Beruna also relates a typical portrayal of "Bluestockings": "[I]hr Haushalt ist in grauenhafter Unordnung, – gegen Mann und Kinder hegen sie eine naturwidrige Gleichgültigkeit, – der Gatte solcher Frauen ist eine Null und spielt neben ihr eine klägliche Rolle" (22). Although this passage is clearly a satire of male anxieties, it also demonstrates that the acquisition of a better social position by women made possible through the admission to higher education would necessarily affect the notion of masculinity as well. Since both genders are constructed as opposites, the strengthening of the woman's position would have to be followed by a simultaneous weakening of male authority in order to preserve the nature of opposites.[152]

Beruna also points out that although some men do feel attracted to smart women, an academically educated and critically thinking woman almost always evokes "die Furcht vorm Blaustrumpf" (19). However, an educated woman would still be accepted in society as long as she would not display greater knowledge or intelligence than men. She illustrates this claim with the following anecdote:

152 Schmersahl advances a similar argument: "Auch wenn im Diskurs über die Geschlechterordnung fast immer 'die' Frau im Mittelpunkt stand, zeigt sich doch, daß Männer letztendlich um sich selbst kreisten und die Verunsicherung ihrer 'Männlichkeit' thematisierten. Die 'Mannweiber' unterminierten nämlich nicht nur die bildungs- und arbeitsmarktpolitische Superiorität des Mannes. Sie stellten auch die Ehre des Mannes und damit *seine* Geschlechtsidentität in Frage, da die 'Vermännlichung' der Frau [...] zu einer 'Verweiblichung' [...] der Männer [...] führe. [...] Viele Autoren der Zeit waren sich darin einig, daß die Frauenemanzipation ursächlich mit der Effeminierung des Mannes zusammenhänge" (327-328). See also Mazón 47 ["Since gender roles in Imperial Germany were defined in opposition to each other, the discussion of the student's masculinity necessarily implies something about contemporary ideas of femininity"] and 94 ["In an era in which gender roles were strictly divided and hierarchical, suggesting that women could do something formerly reserved for men called everything else into question"].

> Herr X erzählt Frau Y von den neuesten Fortschritten der Elektrotechnik; sie hört seinem anregenden Vortrag mit freundlicher Aufmerksamkeit zu. Er ist entzückt von der ungemein liebenswürdigen Dame. Ein anderes Mal will er Frau Z über das Leben der Ameisen unterrichten; nun hat aber diese zufällig vor einigen Tagen einen gemeinverständlichen Aufsatz über die Ameisen gelesen, sie hat reges Interesse für die Natur und schon mehrfach andere Gelegenheit gehabt, sich auf diesem Gebiete zu unterrichten. Kurz – sie weiß das, was der Herr Professor sie lehren will, wie er aus ihren von Klarheit und Verständnis zeugenden Aeußerungen hört. – "Wie gefällt Ihnen Frau Z?" fragt man ihn anderen Tages. "Hm, ist etwas blaustrumpfig angehaucht, hat mehr Vorliebe für die Naturwissenschaften, als mir für das Gedeihen ihres Haushaltes wünschenswerth erscheint. Solche Frauen sind mir unsympathisch, es fehlt ihnen das naiv Weibliche." (Beruna 20-21)

This anecdote demonstrates once again the indissoluble link between the notion of femininity and masculinity as well as the conversely proportional relationship between the two. In order to preserve the alleged male superiority as the main gender characteristic, an "overdeveloped" intellect in women had to be defined as an abnormal feature.

Texts written by men against the participation of women in the medical profession surprisingly often evoke the image of a female with a knife in front of a naked male body. This terrifying fantasy illustrates and magnifies male anxieties about shifting gender roles. Kirchhoff's collection provides a number of examples demonstrating that such a constellation was perceived to be unthinkable. Franz Riegel, for instance, notes the incongruity between the knife and femininity: "Wer jemals die Gelegenheit gehabt hat, Studentinnen im anatomischen Hörsaal zu beobachten, der wird den Eindruck mit sich genommen haben, daß nichts dem Weibe unweiblicher steht, als das anatomische oder chirurgische Messer" (Kirchhoff 77). Gustav Fritsch also draws a similar conclusion: "Die unvermeidliche Brutalität, welche darin liegt, das Messer in einen lebendigen Körper zu stoßen, wirkt beim Manne nicht so verletzend als beim Weibe, wo sie leicht einen abstoßenden Charakter bekommt" (Kirchhoff 46). Johannes Orth cites a situation that is unacceptable to him: "Man denke sich nur die junge Dame im Seziersaal mit Messer und Pincette vor der gänzlich entblößten männlichen Leiche sitzen und Muskeln oder Gefäße und Nerven oder Eingeweide präparieren, [...], - man stelle sich das einmal so recht lebhaft vor [...]" (Kirchhoff 69). Hermann Cohn disapproves on aesthetic grounds: "[…] schön finde ich es […] nicht, wenn eine junge Dame in Gegenwart von Männern auf der Anatomie Leichen zergliedert oder auf der Hautklinik syphilitische Männer untersucht" (Kirchhoff 110).[153] Most of

153 These images are reminiscent of the femmes fatales represented in much of the literature and art of the late nineteenth century such as the biblical heroines Salome, Judith, or Delilah or

these quotations depict a situation in which a female doctor examines the male body. In other words, the woman is in a position of authority and becomes the mediator/producer of specific scientific knowledge[154] about the male body over which she exercises absolute control. Conversely, man is objectified and becomes the passive body without a voice. The woman becomes an autonomous subject, while man becomes the dependent object of her examination. Such a reversal of gender roles was not acceptable because it designated a reversal of power relations.

The female medical student takes on an especially monstrous dimension in an article "Weibliche Ärzte" written by Fritz Wittels (Avicenna) for *Die Fackel.*[155] The article gives the reader a glimpse of what might be called a pathological fear of the female medical student and doctor. Wittels, a Viennese journalist, physician, and student of Freud (Tichy, "Die geschlechtliche Un-Ordnung" 40), tries to explain a woman's desire for medical education as an expression of her perverted sexual drive. He paints a vivid picture of raging and uncontrollable female physicians who use the medical profession to satisfy their perverse urges. He compares female medical students to maenads, demented women in the procession of Dionysus who "were [...] supposed, in their ecstasy, to practice the *sparagmos,* the tearing of living victims to pieces and feasting on their raw flesh" ("Maenad." *Encyclopaedia Britannica*, CD-ROM). Another of his very graphic depictions is a comparison of the female physician to Medea: "in jedem Weibe steckt eine Medea, und Medea war eine Ärztin..." (Avicenna 20). As noted in the introduction, Medea's act of slaying her children in order to take revenge on her lover, Jason, for wanting to marry another woman is, in the traditional telling of the myth, a monstrous deed. By taking lives of her children for the sake of personal vengeance, Medea exceeds, in the nineteeth-century bourgeois imagination, all conceivable social limits. These two symbolic figures, maenad and Medea, demonstrate the nexus of irrationality, murder, sexuality, and perversion that Wittels imposes on the female students and physicians. Moreover, by stating that

---

female figures modeled on them like Rosa Fröhlich in Heinrich Mann's *Professor Unrath* and Gerda von Rinnlingen in Thomas Mann's *Der kleine Herr Friedemann.* For a secondary literature regarding representations of femininity in fin-de-siècle literature see Weiershausen 11.

154 Weiershausen points out that the fact that the university was a place of knowledge production was one of the reasons for the debate about women's admission to higher education being so heated (29-30). She writes: "Vor dem Hintergrund einer strukturellen Ausgrenzung der Frau als dem 'Anderen' und ihrem damit einhergehenden Status als Objekt der Diskurse mußte ihr Eintritt in die universitäre Welt die bisher gültigen Ordnungssysteme grundlegend in Frage stellen" (30). Weiershausen also emphasizes "das männliche Wissensmonopol und die damit zusammenhängende Definitionsmacht" (58).

155 Tichy discusses this article extensively in "Die geschlechtliche Un-Ordnung" 40-42. She uses it as an example illustrating what she calls "[d]ie Verpathologisierung weiblicher Intellektualität" (40). According to her, Wittels' article is noteworthy because of "seiner erbarmungslosen Fülle an geschlechtsspezifischen Ideologemen (40).

"in jedem Weibe steckt eine Medea," Wittels hints at a latent pathological dimension in all women, a quite common view in nineteenth-century Western medicine, as demonstrated by Schmersahl in her study, *Medizin und Geschlecht.*[156]

According to Wittels, there is only one principle that governs a woman's life: the seduction of man ("die Anlockung des Mannes") (Avicenna 10). A woman's pursuit of a medical education is driven by this principle as well. However, in the case of women who do not aspire to become physicians, this principle manifests itself in normal sexual behavior. Female medical students and doctors, on the contrary, suffer from hysteria or at least have "ein bißchen Anlage zur Hysterie" (Avicenna 12) and exhibit abnormal sexual behavior as a result. A manifestation of such abnormal sexual behavior is a quest for an academic career: "Denn das hysterische Weib hat die geheimnisvolle Fähigkeit, seinen Sexualwillen vom Sexualziel abzuziehen und auf die Tätigkeit zu lenken, in die es sich gerade verrannt hat" (Avicenna 11).[157] As a consequence of the displaced sexual desire, female students exhibit what he calls "der [...] wollüstige Fleiß" (Avicenna 12). He characterizes a pursuit of a medical career by women as follows:

> Es ist ein geiler, im bürgerlichen und wohl auch im metaphysischen Sinne unsittlicher Fleiß, das Weib absolviert in Form von Wissenschaft sein Sexualleben vor allen Augen, es ist ein maßloses, bacchanistisches Sichausleben, denn Furcht und Scham, die das normale Weib hemmen, fallen hier weg; es ist eine öffentliche Liebe, von der niemand nichts weiß. (Avicenna 12)[158]

In addition to the displaced sexual drive channeled through the realm of science, female students seduce their male colleagues in order to satisfy their urges in a physical way. The female principle becomes now "die aggressive Art der Anlockung" (Avicenna 14). Wittels' rhetoric transforms these women into aggressive sexual predators whose aim is to corrupt and enslave male students: "Die Gefahr ist groß, daß ein Student mit der ganzen Hartnäckigkeit der ersten Liebe sich in ein Scheusal vergafft, nur weil es ihm immer um die Nase streicht [...]. Das Eindringen des Weibes ins Laboratorium fühlt auch der schüchterne Liebhaber als Angebot, und einmal im Netz, zappelt er lange" (Avicenna 13).[159]

The image of a female physician is even more terrifying than the one of the female student. Now the sexual perversity manifests itself in the struggle for power: "[...] jedermann im Saale muß die Frau Doktor als Herrscherin anerkennen, sonst gibt es Krach. Wir haben es mit der infantilen Form der Herrschsucht zu tun, wie sie sich etwa in einem Häuptling der Dahomeyneger zeigt, der täglich

156 Schmersahl demonstrated that in many medical texts of the nineteenth century femininity was equated with sickness. See Schmersahl, for example, 105-106; 113; 278; 307.

157 Also qtd. in Tichy, "Die geschlechtliche Un-Ordnung" 41.

158 Also qtd. in Tichy, "Die geschlechtliche Un-Ordnung" 41.

159 Also qtd. in Tichy, "Die geschlechtliche Un-Ordnung" 42.

eigenhändig ein paar Untertanen köpft, um sich an seiner Machtfülle zu weiden" (Avicenna 18). The principle of seduction in conjunction with the desire for power would have terrifying consequences for patients who, being at the mercy of the female doctor, would become the target of her unpredictable cruelty: "Besser noch möchte ein Mann, der eine Operateurin durch seine Gleichgültigkeit beleidigt hat, unter ihrem Messer davon kommen, als eine Frau, die neben der Ärztin glücklicher um Mannesgunst gebuhlt hat. Die Ärztin wird der Nebenbuhlerin bei der Operation lockere Darmnähte setzen, daß sie stirbt [...]" (Avicenna 19). In addition, women having access to vulnerable (for example, paralyzed) men would only assault and humiliate them because a healthy man would never allow himself to be examined by a female doctor: "[...] ein Mann sollte sich vor einem Weibe und für ein Weib entblößen können, von ihm besehen, betastet, behorcht werden: mit Ausschluß der Sexualität. [...] Er schämt sich vor dem Weibe; nicht weil er sich entblößen soll, sondern weil es so geschehen soll, als wäre er impotent und exhibitioniere" (Avicenna 16).[160] In this context, a claim made by the feminist psychoanalyst Karen Horney about the foundation of masculinity seems to explain, at least partially, Wittels' antagonism towards female physicians. Horney's paper "The Dread of Woman" published in the *International Journal of Psycho-analysis* in 1932 "crystallized two important points: the extent to which adult masculinity is built on over-reactions to femininity, and the connection of the making of masculinity with the subordination of women" (Connell 11).[161]

3.3 Eduard Albert and the Lack of Scientific Objectivity

Eduard Albert, a Viennese professor of medicine and a fanatical opponent of the admission of women to medical schools, perceives the emergence of a new female type as highly undesirable and as carrying a number of negative consequences for the whole society:

> Das bisherige Naturwesen soll Culturwesen werden. Das ist ein Plan, der die Struktur der Menschheit umändern soll. Die bisherige Einheit, das Element der Menschheit ist das Menschenpaar: der Mann und das Weib. Ein zweiatomiges Molekül. In diesem Molekül binden sich zwei verschiedene Atome M and W. Nun soll das W ersetzt

160 Partly also qtd. in Tichy, "Die geschlechtliche Un-Ordnung" 42.

161 Connell summarizes Horney's argument as follows: "For Horney, fear of the mother is more deep-seated and more energetically repressed than fear of the castrating father. The vagina itself is the symbolic center of the process. Boys' feelings of inadequacy lead them to withdraw emotional energy from the mother and focus it on themselves and their genitals – thus preparing the ground for castration anxiety. Later reactions among men are fuelled by these emotions. Among them are the tendency to choose socially inferior women and love objects, and the habit of actively undermining women's self-respect [...]" (11).

> werden durch ein anderes W, durch W', durch das Weib der Zukunft. (8)[162]

As indicated by this quotation, W'-type that would potentially replace the natural woman (W-type) is perceived as a dangerous mutation that could lead to a new social model. However, Albert claims that such a mutation is ultimately not possible. Even if some women could develop their intellect if subjected to higher education, they would not be able to pass these intellectual qualities on to their daughters. Educated women would only pass the positive traits on to their sons. Moreover, Albert maintains that women are not able to inherit the intellectual aptitude from their fathers due to the limits imposed by the female brain. Consequently a permanent change in the intellectual capacity of the female sex is not possible (Albert 9).

Albert's pamphlet *Die Frauen und das Studium der Medicin* offers, however, a highly misogynistic caricature of gender roles and achievements rather than an objective scientific exploration. Due to its obvious misogyny and lack of scientific support, Albert's text was very critically received in the academic community. In an article published in *Die Frauenbewegung* in February 1896, Minna Cauer notes that in Vienna "Prof. Alberts Broschüre wie eine Bombe wirkte" (26). Similarily, Marianne Hainisch points out that

> die masslos heftigen Angriffe Hofrat Professor Alberts [...] [entfesselten] binnen wenig Monaten eine Anzahl Protestversammlungen und drei Gegenschriften. Auch wurde die Streitfrage wochenlang zum Gesprächsthema in Kreisen, die sich bis dahin nicht für die Frauenbestrebungen interessiert hatten, so dass in den letzten 25 Jahren nichts so sehr die Frauenbewegung gefördert hat, als die Aussprüche tiefster Missachtung, die der Essay des Gelehrten enthielt. ("Geschichte" 176)[163]

Unlike Waldeyer's speech and publication of 1888, Albert's text actually helped women gain support for higher education. Hainisch connects its publication with a

162 Albert's use of M and W is reminiscent of Otto Weininger's work *Geschlecht und Charakter.*

163 Hainisch names three direct responses to Albert: Dr. E. Hannak, *Professor Alberts Essay: Die Frauen und das Studium der Medizin* (1895); Dr. M. Kronfeld *Die Frauen und die Medizin. Professor Albert zur Antwort* (1895); and a text by herself, *Seherinnen, Hexen und die Wahnvorstellungen über das Weib im 19. Jahrhundert* (1896). In addition to these texts, Sveistrup and Zahn-Harnack refer to a response to Albert by E. Ehrlich, *Zur Frage des Frauenstudiums*. Finally, Albert's pamphlet generated additional responses by Minna Cauer, "Die Wissenschaft und die Frauen," Irma von Troll-Borostyáni, "Heilfrauen – statt Ärztinnen," Helene Lange, "Professor Albert und das medizinische Studium der Frauen," and Eliza Ichenhaeuser in her book *Die Ausnahmestellung Deutschlands in Sachen des Frauenstudiums* (See Works Cited).

lively debate in the Austrian parliament regarding the issue of higher education for women, in which most of the parliamentarians supported the cause ("Geschichte" 176). Hainisch also refers to a number of successes on the legislative level:

> Noch in demselben Jahre, am 15. April 1896, erschien das Verordnungsblatt des Ministeriums für Kultus und Unterricht, welches bestimmte, dass die Nostrifikation der von Frauen im Auslande erworbenen medizinischen Doktorendiplome gestattet sei; eine grössere Anzahl ausserordentlicher Hörerinnen wurde an der medizinischen Fakultät inskribiert; es wurde sogar ein Stipendium für eine ordentliche Hörerin der Medizin an der Wiener Universität gestattet. ("Geschichte" 176)

Albert's text was further criticized because it did not bring any new arguments to bear on the debate about women's pursuit of medicine. Throughout his pamphlet, Albert emphasizes the lack of reason and intellect in women. The text consists of a number of derogatory and contemptuous epithets directed towards women including an anecdote about one of Albert's female patients with which the author tries to illustrate the woman's lack of logical thought. For Albert, women are one-dimensional beings without any higher aspirations: "Es ist immer das ewige 'Ich', das autonome Protoplasma, was im Weibe zur Geltung kommt; der ewige dumme Wille zum Leben [...]" (Albert 15).[164] Throughout his pamphlet, Albert emphasizes the distinction between nature (woman) and culture (man). This dichotomy parallels the split between the private and public realms, in which woman is limited to the reproductive function at home, and man is unrestricted within the public space.[165]

Although Albert does not contribute anything new to the discussion about women's education, his text is important because it sets up a new stage in the public debate in which physicians no longer attempt to provide a scientific basis of gender inequality. Bischoff and Waldeyer, although unquestionably influenced by their personal misogyny, used scientific data and referred to research regarding the capacity of the human brain. Although in a highly manipulative way, they still tried to provide a scientific validation for their claims. Albert clearly undermines his own medical and scientific authority by letting his personal views take absolute control of what is supposed to be an objective scientific voice.[166] Cauer dismisses Albert's text as follows: "Fast ist man geneigt anzunehmen, daß Prof. Albert in

164 Also qtd. in Tichy, "Die geschlechtliche Un-Ordnung" 32.

165 The binary opposition between culture and nature and the critique thereof will be discussed in Chapter Five.

166 According to Tichy, Albert's text "demonstriert in paradigmatischer Reinheit, was die mit wissenschaftlichem Anspruch vorgetragene Ablehnung des Frauenstudiums charakterisiert [...]," that is, lack of logic and the blurred boundary between science and ideology ("Die geschlechtliche Un-Ordnung" 33).

einer tief inneren Entrüstung diese Ausfälle gegen die Frauen 'hingeworfen' hat, weil er fühlt, daß 'trotz alledem und alledem' die Frauen mit Erfolg in das medizinische Studium eindringen werden" (26). She makes it clear that due to the lack of scientific evidence regarding the alleged female inferiority and due to the demonstrated successes of female students and physicians, Albert and the like are forced to move beyond science in order to ridicule women's attempts to enter the medical profession. By so doing, however, the opponents of female education lose their credibility. Anne Fausto-Sterling argues that scientifically "unanswerable questions drop out of the realm of science altogether, entering instead that of philosophy and morality" (*Myths of Gender* 8). Indeed, many medical doctors shifted the focus of the discussion from the realm of science to the realm of morality while arguing against female education. After it became clear that women were able to pursue a medical or other academic career successfully, authors trying to discredit women's ability to think moved their explorations to the realm of philosophy. Otto Weininger and Georg Groddeck are causes in point.

Regardless of whether the texts discrediting a woman's ability to think and pursue an academic education are of a scientific or philosophical nature, they all seem to be driven by a male supremacist ideology. Although some methods, means, and argumentation change in the course of history, the underlying motivation is always the same. Hainisch makes this ideological foundation very clear when she places Albert's text on a straight axis leading from the pre-modern witch-hunt to the modern day attempt to keep women excluded from academic education. She recognizes that a certain paradigm shift mirrored the transition from the pre-modern to the modern era in terms of gender relations; specifically, scientific authority replaced church authority and the witch transformed into a female physician. In the context of the witch-craze, Hainisch speaks of "Phantasieverbrechen und Phantasieverbrecherinnen für deren Schuld kein Beweis erbracht werden konnte" (*Seherinnen* 12). The foundation of the pre-modern belief in witchcraft lies outside of a scientifically verifiable realm. Similarily, the alleged female intellectual inferiority cannot be scientifically proven. Hainisch further calls attention to the financial factor that certainly influenced the persistence with which certain individuals pointed their fingers at the alleged witches since such a denunciation frequently involved a monetary compensation. Respectively, as I argued in Chapters One and Two, the fear of competition on the job market was an important element of the resistance towards the admission of women to medical schools. Finally, the fervor demonstrated by the Inquisition is paralleled by the zeal displayed by the opponents of women's entrance into academia. According to Hainisch, Albert shows as much fanaticism in his convictions as the two Dominican priests who wrote the infamous *Malleus Maleficarum*:[167] "[..] dieses Temperamentvolle in seinen [Alberts] Auseinandersetzungen zeigt, daß auch der

167 *Malleus Maleficarum* was "the standard handbook on witchcraft" that appeared in 1486 and was written by Johann Sprenger and Heinrich Kraemer ("Malleus Maleficarum." *Encyclopaedia Britannica*, CD-ROM).

hervorragende Arzt den Spuren der Dominikaner folgt" (*Seherinnen* 17). Hence, she stresses the ideological foundation of Albert's pamphlet that relegates it to the realm of fanatical distortions of reality.

3.4 The Female Body as an Object of Aesthetic and Sensual Pleasure

Fausto-Sterling argues that even at the end of the twentieth century "research about sex differences frequently contains gross procedural errors" and suggests that "scientists themselves emerge as cultural products" (*Myths of Gender* 8-9). She further claims that "[i]n analyzing male/female differences these scientists peer through the prism of everyday culture, using the colors so separated to highlight their questions, design their experiments, and interpret their results. More often than not their hidden agendas, non-conscious and thus unarticulated, bear strong resemblances to broader social agendas" (*Myths of Gender* 9). Almost one hundred years earlier, many women made similar claims in the context of the debate about women's admission to medical schools. They emphasized a strong connection among the scientific research regarding gender differences, arguments against medical education, and the nineteenth-century perception of women as objects of aesthetic or sensual pleasure for heterosexual men.

Nineteenth-century male culture and science created woman as a secondary being whose existence was largely defined in terms of male pleasure and/or reproduction. As Mayreder noted: "[...] das Weib [ist] nur ein Mittel zum Zweck – erstens zur Befriedigung des Mannes, zweitens zur Hervorhebung des Mannes, der das Endziel aller Veranstaltungen sowohl der Natur wie des Staates bildet" ("Die schöne Weiblichkeit" 120). Since both male sexual pleasure and the female reproductive functions were popularly believed to diminish as a result of women's participation in higher education, it is not surprising that many scientists and other opponents of female medical education tried to provide suitable evidence or even manipulate existing scientific research to make it fit their agenda. Mayreder contends that there are two characteristics that constitute what is perceived as femininity: "beauty" and "weakness." She claims: "Man wird unter den kanonischen Vorzügen der schönen Weiblichkeit kaum einen finden, der nicht unter diese beiden Kategorien zu reihen wäre" ("Die schöne Weiblichkeit" 121). The gender-specific perception of these two categories perpetuates female exclusion from the public space, in general, and from the medical education, in particular. The beauty/physicality of a married middle-class woman is reserved only for her husband and cannot be exposed to the public view. The alleged bodily and mental weakness condemns her to the private realm and to dependency on male "protection."

Mayreder also accentuates the status of the female body as an aesthetic object. While genius and ethics are entirely male domains, women's existence is limited to the aesthetic aspect. As she points out "Anmuth und Schönheit [sind] das Genie des Weibes" and "die Stelle welche beim Manne Ethik vertritt, [wird] beim Weibe durch die Aesthetik eingenommen" ("Die schöne Weiblichkeit" 121).

At the same time, she makes it very clear that this "aesthetic genius" of women is not creative. Rather, Mayreder argues, women are generally defined as passive aesthetic material that has yet to be molded by men. According to Mayreder, the notion of a woman who cannot exist without a man, because she has to be created by him, is rooted in the male "subjective erotische Phantasie" ("Die schöne Weiblichkeit" 122). In other words it is not grounded in reality, but rather it is a creation of the male imagination: "Die Vorstellung, ein Wesen mit bestimmten angeborenen Eigenschaften – und auch das willenschwächste Weib ist ein solches Wesen – nach eigener Willkür erst 'schaffen' zu können, stammt nicht aus der Beobachtung wirklicher Vorgänge; sie gehört unter jene Illusionen, an denen die psychosexuellen Beziehungen der Menschen so reich sind" ("Die schöne Weiblichkeit" 122). In the context of Mayreder's article, I argue that higher education of women would cancel out the male fantasies about "creating the woman" according to certain expectations because it would give women tools (for example, critical thinking, knowledge, independence) to "create themselves" as independent beings. Consequently, they would become more than "[e]in schwacher Abklatsch" (Dohm, *Emancipation* 178) of men. The notion of woman as an aesthetic potential that comes into being through men reinforces the perception that women are the passive objects of male pleasure.

Morgenstern addresses the apparent male anxiety regarding women's entrance into the academic fields by raising the following question: "Warum befürchten die Männer, daß die Frau durch das Studium ungenießbar werden [sic] und an Achtung verlieren wird, während sie selbst durch ihr Wissen eine bevorzugte Stellung in der Gesellschaft einnehmen [...]" (18-19). As indicated by this quotation, a higher social status combined with knowledge and financial independence would cause a shift in woman's position in relation to men. Instead of being forced to be perpetually dependent on men, women could enter the public arena as equals and as self-reliant individuals. Hence, Morgenstern implies that the image of a strong woman necessitates a re-evaluation of gender standards including a redefinition of masculinity.[168]

Dohm, as well, exposes the politics of the female body as a driving force behind arguments against female medical education. She sees Bischoff's views as representative of the male notion of femininity at the end of the nineteenth century and argues that such convictions are rooted in the popular perception of gender roles. Dohm further asserts that under the male gaze women are perceived exclusively as bodies expected to provide aesthetic or sensual pleasure to heterosexual men. Any act that is believed to diminish such an experience of pleasure, for example, the study of medicine, is defined as unfeminine and received with antagonism. For this reason, Dohm argues, academic education is understood as "ein ästhetisches Malheur für die Frau" (*Emancipation* 173). Referring to the medical profession, Bischoff highlights the male perspective on femininity and claims in

168 See footnote 152.

his pamphlet that in a female physician, a patient would only see a sexual being and would not be able to perceive her as a medical doctor:

> Wenn man an dem Krankenbette [...] mit Zittern und Zagen und zugleich mit Hoffnung auf Hülfe, Rettung und Trost dem Arzte entgegensieht, dann kann ich mir ohnmöglich denken, daß *das frisierte Haar* und *die rauschenden Röcke* einer Frau dem Kranken diese Hoffnung und diesen Trost bringen werden. (36; emphasis added)

In this context, Bischoff contrasts the female body with "male authority," both being mutually exclusive. On the basis of male authority and intellect, a patient seeks help, hope, and comfort from a male physician. A female doctor would not be able to transcend her bodily nature and would not evoke trust in a male patient who, according to Bischoff, perceives women only through the prism of their sexuality. In line with this reasoning, women can evoke only an aesthetic ("frisiertes Haar") or sensory ("rauschende Röcke") experience based on their outward appearance, while men evoke trust and hope based on their internal authority. Dohm makes us aware of the arbitrariness of such connotations:

> Der Herr Professor können sich nicht denken, daß *frisiertes Haar* und *rauschende Röcke* dem Kranken Trost und Hofnung bringen. Das glaube ich auch nicht; ich glaube aber auch nicht, daß *knarrende Stiefel, hohe Zylinderhüte* oder *Kahlköpfe* Trost und Hoffnung zu bringen im Stande sind. Auch daß die Anmuth einer wohlfrisierten Perrücke Trost und Hoffnung bringe, muß ich bezweifeln. *(Emancipation* 157; emphasis added)

Dohm points out that Bischoff consciously singles out the physical aspect of the female body while focusing on the spiritual and mental dimension in men. She calls attention to the physical dimension of the male body as well in order to show that Bischoff not only acts upon gender stereotypes of the time, but also caricatures the image of the male and female doctor.

A similar exclusive focus on the sexualized female body seems to be informing Bischoff's hostility towards a potential pregnancy of the female physician: "Wie interessant, passend und würdevoll muß es nicht sein, die Frau Ärztin sich mit schwangerem Leibe am Krankenbette und Operationstische umherbewegen zu sehen!?" (Bischoff 38-39). Dohm indicates that the sight of a pregnant physician would disturb only those men for whom a woman's primary role is to deliver aesthetic or sensual pleasure and who perceive women exclusively as decorative beings. Dohm implies that the sight of a pregnant woman negates expectations of visual pleasure imposed on the female body by heterosexual men. She contends: "[D]ie Erscheinung einer Frau, die guter Hoffnung ist, verletzt das Schönheitsgefühl ihrer Umgebung, stört ihr ästhetisches Behagen" (*Emancipation*

139). Bischoff's aversion to the sight of a pregnant woman only confirms the ornamental status of the female body in men's eyes. Similarily, another female activist, Dr. H. Paul[169] points out: "Für viele ist eine schwangere Frau nur eine komische Figur oder ein unästhetischer Anblick und die Zielscheibe ihrer abscheulichen Witze" (25). Dohm indicates that such a perspective is very limited and determined solely by the male sexual drive. On the other side of the spectrum are women and children who, unlike men, do not pay any attention to the aesthetic aspects of the female doctor's body (*Emancipation* 139-40).

Dohm emphasizes Bischoff's focus on the surface of the female body as she refers to "die schönen Körperlinien" (*Emancipation* 139). The male gaze reduces women to their bodies and does not acknowledge their intellectual or spiritual dimensions. Dohm points out that Bischoff places much value on bodily aesthetics but only with respect to the female body: "[M]üßten nicht von diesem ästhetischen Gesichtspunkt aus auch alle Männer, die sich von der Normalgestalt des Apollo von Belvedere um so und so viel Linien böswillig entfernt haben, aller öffentlichen Aemter beraubt und ihrer ärztlichen Funktionen enthoben werden?" (*Emancipation* 140). According to Bischoff, men do not have to conform to any aesthetic principles. However, laws and regulations, Dohm asserts, should be applied uniformly to men and women.

Like Dohm, Binder also makes it very explicit that the male determination to exclude women from academic education is fueled by the fear of women losing their feminine traits. She paraphrases Dr. Kaiser,[170] one of the opponents of higher medical education for women, as follows: "Alles, was die Frau dem Manne begehrenswert macht, geht unwiederbringlich verloren, wenn sie sich Berufsformen zuwendet, die eine höhere geistige Ausbildung erfordern, und dieses 'Alles' nennt Dr. Kaiser mit dem vielbergenden Namen 'Weiblichkeit'" (Binder 27). She further critically analyzes this particular position by stating: "[Es] wird [...] schwer fallen, der darin versteckten Drohung, der Mann könnte unter Umständen aufhören des Weibes zu begehren, mit unsatirischem Ernst zu begegnen" (Binder 27). Unlike Dohm, however, who deems male desires regarding women's appearance and personality to be an expression of unjustifiable egoism, Binder validates them by arguing that women's participation in higher education could not possibly change what is perceived as femininity and what is desirable to men. On the contrary, according to Binder, female qualities, such as "die Geduld, [...] das sanfte Wort, die dienende Liebe" (Binder 28) are needed in the medical field. Hence, they would flourish and not disappear. Binder further describes the conventional male expectations of so-called femininity:

169 Her first name is unknown.

170 She does not identify him by his first name but refers to his article "Ueber die Zulassung der Frauen zu den höheren Berufsformen des Mannes." Beil. Zur Allg. Zt. 18. Febr. 1891, Nr. 49 (Binder 15).

> Was der Mann beim Weibe sucht, ist Freude. Freude, Lebensanmut und Lebensbequemlichkeit. Daß diese ihm gewahrt bleiben, darauf steht sein Verlangen, [...]. Die sicherste Garantie hierfür vermutet er darin, daß auf der Frauen Seite jene ganze Summen von Eigenschaften, die man gewöhnlich unter "Weiblichkeit" begreift, immer in reichlicher Vertretung gefunden werde. Die Fügsamkeit vor allem und die Geduld, das Bedürfnis aufzublicken und zu verehren, [...] das sanfte Schweigen und das sanfte Wort, die dienende Liebe. Selbst unser weibliches Schönheitsideal ist großenteils dahin berechnet. Der schlanke Leib, der leicht umfasst und festgehalten werden kann, die weichen Formen, die nirgends verletzen und wenig Ellbogenraum beanspruchen, die kleine Hand, die wenigstens wehrlos scheint, der zarte Fuß, der auch die Fliehende nicht weithin trägt. (28)

Dohm and Binder, as intellectuals, use different strategies to negotiate new roles for women. Dohm refuses altogether to accept the notion that the female body's primary function is to provide men with aesthetic and sensual pleasure. Women's position in society defined only in terms of male desire is intolerable to her. Binder, alternatively, validates male claims by stating: "[D]er Mann steht auf dem Boden seines natürlichen Rechtes, wenn er von diesen guten und hübschen Dingen [see the quotation above], die soviel zu seiner irdischen Glückseligkeit beizutragen vermögen, kein Jota einbüßen will" (Binder 28). However, she tries to negotiate an additional purpose for the above-mentioned female qualities: "[E]in guter Teil der vorerwähnten Tugenden und Eigenschaften fände eben in deren künftigem Beruf vorzügliche Verwendung" (Binder 28). In addition to serving men and making their existence more pleasurable, women should utilize their feminine characteristics, for instance by working in the medical profession. Morgenstern uses another strategy. She calls attention to the benefits that men would gain from having an educated wife: "Und wird es nicht vielmehr besser im Haushalte werden, wenn die Frau in demselben ihre wissenschaftlichen Kenntnisse und Erfahrungen verwertet?" (Morgenstern 8-19). Both Binder and Morgenstern attempt to convince their readers that an academic education would not diminish feminine characteristics. In so doing both writers validate male claims to the desirable female body. Dohm, on the contrary, exposes the double standards of such argumentation. She implies that none of the opponents of the admission of women to universities would admit that it is predominantly the female body that is at stake in this struggle. For her, however, this is obviously the case: "Wäre es aber wahr, daß [...] die Zunahme des Wissens bei ihr [der Frau] eine Abnahme weiblicher Anmuth bedingte, so würde diese schadhafte Grazie doch nur ein Verlust sein für die *Augen* der Männer und nicht für ihre *Seele*" (Dohm, *Emancipation* 176). Dohm exposes the main function women were expected to fulfill, namely, satisfaction of male desires for aesthetic and sensual pleasure.

In addition, Dohm shows the relative value of conventional judgments and expectations regarding femininity. The same quality can be simultaneously perceived as both feminine and unfeminine, existent and non-existent in women, depending on the context. Through the prism of the standards of physical beauty of the time, for instance, women were expected not to exhibit any physical strength.[171] Arguing against female medical education, Bischoff asserts that women do not possess the required strength to succeed in this position: "[M]an denke sich eine grössere chirurgische Operation, Amputation, Exarticulation, Steinschnitt etc. etc., welches Mannweib würde dazu gehören, um die nöthigen Kräfte aufzutreiben!" (36). In addition, Bischoff asserts that women lack "Sicherheit und Herrschaft über die nothwendigen Bewegungen" (36) to perform any kind of surgery. However, Dohm provides examples such as the performance of a ballet-dancer or a "Seiltänzerin" to prove this statement to be wrong. These women have more strength and precision than most of the professors of medicine. In addition, such women are praised as the apogee of femininity: "Entzückend weiblich erscheinen diese Damen den Männern [...], und das: '*Anathema sit*' verwandelt sich bei ihrem Anblick in ein Wonneschmunzeln. Diese Frauen leisten das Höchste, was Männer von den Frauen fordern: *sie amusiren*!" (Dohm, *Emancipation* 126). As Dohm indicates, Bischoff's reasoning is based on the conviction that the sole purpose of a woman's existence is to deliver pleasure and entertainment to men. If a woman tries to use her talents in a different realm, she is branded a "Mannweib." Morgenstern advances an argument similar to the one presented by Dohm: "Aber niemals haben Männer verboten, diese Künste [Seiltanzen und Reiten], die zu sehen ihnen ein Vergnügen bereiten, obgleich sie entgegengesetzt den Geschlechtseigenschaften der Frau sind, die man von ihr verlangt" (Morgenstern 20).

Bischoff argues that there is a connection between the acquisition of knowledge and the deterioration of the female body. According to him, education creates in girls "tiefe und lebenslänglich nachwirkende Beeinträchtigung" (21). He contends that young women exposed to learning suffer from physical and psychological impairments: "Sie haben die Gesundheit, Unbefangenheit, Liebenswürdigkeit, Heiterkeit, Anstelligkeit und Bereitwilligkeit der weiblichen Jugend verloren, sind kränklich, voller fremdartiger Ansprüche" (Bischoff 21). Dohm reverses his equation and argues that not education, but precisely its opposite, the lack of appropriate intellectual stimulation, creates sickly and neurotic women. Girls are not encouraged to develop their intellect and have to participate in mind-numbing activities instead, such as superficial social interactions, balls, and mechanical household chores. The upbringing of upper- and middle-class women cripples them intellectually. Their minds do not receive adequate guidance and as a result, they drift into the realm of fantasy and illusions. The mind's perpetual slumber and

171 Dijkstra refers to this nineteenth-century phenomenon as "The Cult of Invalidism" (*Idols of Perversity* 25). For a discussion of a representation of this phenomenon in art see Dijkstra, *Idols of Perversity* 25-118.

inactivity causes psychological and physical damage in women (Dohm, *Emancipation* 147- 48).

Dohm points out that an academic pursuit is often seen as "ein ästhetisches Unglück" because it is believed to cause women a loss of their visual and sexual appeal (*Emancipation* 168). In the male imagination, thinking and knowledgeable women turn into deformed creatures. Hence, an over-developed intellect in women is perceived as an abnormal feature that causes the female body to deteriorate:

> Mit dem Begriff einer starkgeistigen, d.h. denkenden und wissenden Frau verbindet man gern die Vorstellung von *harten Zügen, einer langen Nase*, Stiefeln mit Randsohlen, Charakterkanten und einer, wenn auch unverschuldeten, so doch unerfreulichen Aeltlichkeit. Besonders phantasiereiche männliche Gemüther neigen auch zur Annahme eines *kleinen Schnauzbartes* und *einer Rabenstimme*. (Dohm, *Emancipation* 174; emphasis added)

Dohm argues that this anticipated female degeneration is merely a construct of the male imagination. She relies on historical precedents to prove this theory to be wrong. She cites examples of highly educated women who did not lose any part of their femininity, for example, an Italian woman, the "göttliche [...] Isotta," who had to cover her face with a veil while holding law lectures at the university "um die Zuhörer nicht durch ihre Schönheit zu verwirren" (Dohm, *Emancipation* 174). Dohm dismisses the connection between a developed intellect and the unpleasing appearance in women as groundless and unjustifiable. Furthermore, she claims that this hypothesis was invented by men: "Daß Grazie, edle Weiblichkeit und wissenschaftliche Erkenntniss einander ausschließen, ist einer der burleskesten Einfälle, die je ein männlicher Denkerkopf ersonnen" (Dohm, *Emancipation* 176).

As opposed to the notion of knowledge capable of visually deforming the female body, Marie Raschke critiques the concept of the female body not being able to "digest" knowledge. In her article entitled "Wissen verdummt," Raschke calls attention to statements made by two parliamentarians regarding female education:

> Herr Abgeordneter Irmer meint: "In unseren Mädchenschulen wird an Wissen viel zu viel geleistet. – Das Bestreben, die Bildung der Mädchen quantitativ zu erweitern, bringt eine große Gefahr in sich. Wir dürfen nicht Puppen erziehen, welche mit ihrem großen Wissen später nichts anfangen können, sonst geht das ganze Gemütsleben unseres Volkes verloren." (51)

Another member of parliament argued similarly: "Das Übermaß von Wissen ist nur ein Hindernis für die Mädchen; je mehr Wissen man ihnen einpfropft, desto dümmer werden sie" (qtd. in Raschke, "Wissen verdummt" 51). According to these statements, women are, indeed, not able to process an excess of knowledge and if subjected to higher education they would completely lose their already limited mental power.

On the basis of my analysis of the rhetorical strategies used by the opponents of women's education, as compared to those in Dohm's book and Raschke's article, I propose that knowledge is generally perceived by opponents as a foreign organism invading the female body and deforming it. It becomes a gender-specific illness that always produces damage on the internal and external level. The effects might range from the deterioration of the female reproductive organs, the weakening of general health, to hysteria, and the decrease of mental faculties. The internal damage sometimes manifests itself in external symptoms such as loss of the feminine body features. Hence, universities and medical schools become institutions spreading the "knowledge-disease." Therefore, keeping women away from higher education makes them less susceptible to the "infection." Consequently, arguments against the admission of women to the universities and medical schools are framed as motivated by the concern for the "women's own good"[172] and the necessity to preserve the health of the nation. Women have to prove that they are immune to the "disease" and able to remain feminine. In such cases, they would even be permitted to attend academic lectures from time to time. Anna Beruna ironically illustrates this reasoning by the following example:

> Gern wird ihr [der Frau] der Besuch des Vortrages vergeben, wenn sie hernach sagt: "Ach, ich habe so vieles nicht verstanden, bitte, Herr Doktor erklären sie mir doch noch einmal dies oder das" – oder wenn sie gar mit schelmischem Lächeln hinzu setzt: "Nein lassen Sie das Erklären nur lieber, ich vergesse es ja doch wieder!" Aber schlimm, sehr schlimm ist es, wenn sie Anderen das Gehörte mit Verständnis zu berichten weiß, und wenn dabei ihr Gedächtnis nicht einmal der Nachhilfe des anwesenden Herrn Doktors bedarf!" (21)

Here, again, a woman has to demonstrate that she is not "susceptible" to knowledge or critical thinking that could potentially diminish her femininity.

As noted in Chapter One, individual professors could give or withdraw their permission regarding women's participation in lectures and seminars at any time. Consequently, women were dependent entirely on the personal convictions of individual professors whose lectures they wanted to attend. Morgenstern calls attention to an additional factor that could potentially become decisive in such situations: the status of the female body as an object of aesthetic or sensual pleasure. The admission of women to selected lectures would not be based on their intellectual qualification, but rather it would be granted according to "dem

172 See the title of a book by Barbara Ehrenreich and Deirdre English, *For Her Own Good. 150 Years of the Experts' Advice to Women*. New York: Doubleday, 1978.

Ermessen einzelner Professoren, wie ihnen die Studentin gefällt" (Morgenstern 21). She inquires:

> Und welchen Maßstab werden die Professoren alsdann an die Jüngerin der Wissenschaft anlegen? Im Allgemeinen ist es ja bekannt, daß selbst die gelehrten Herren der Schönheit und weiblichen Anmut nicht widerstehen können, während Hässlichkeit und körperliche Gebrechen sie abstoßen. Wohin würde es nun führen, wenn die Zuhörerschaft der Frauen von dem *willkürlichen* Ermessen jedes Professors abhängen würde? (Morgenstern 21)

Dohm also addresses this issue. She points out that Bischoff and another opponent of female higher education, a philosophy professor from Bonn,[173] declare support for admitting a few attractive women to selected lectures. Dohm quotes both professors to the effect that they consider women to be objects of aesthetic (if not sexual) pleasure. Regarding the idea of admitting selected female students to the academic lectures, Bischoff writes: "Warum sollte man nicht (wo es sich nicht um ein Prinzip handelt) da und dort einer *interessanten*, intelligenten, auch *hübschen* Frau gestatten, eine Vorlesung über irgend eine unverfängliche Disciplin zu besuchen?" (qtd. in Dohm, *Emancipation* 53). The philosophy professor shares Bischoff's opinion: "Einzelne Männer sind selten im Stande gewesen, einer lernbegierigen und *nicht unliebenswürdigen* Schülerin ihre Theilnahme und Hülfe zu versagen" (Dohm, *Emancipation* 53). Such declarations exemplify the connection between the educational politics and the status of the female body as a source of male aesthetic and sensual pleasure. Dohm concludes that the attitudes of men opposing female higher education are fueled by a "lieblose, erzdespotische, schauderhaft egoistische Gesinnung" (*Emancipation* 54) that privileges male satisfaction. If this were not the case, these professors would advocate the admission of precisely the "Häßlichsten und Unliebenswürdigsten" because these women are less likely to marry and therefore more likely forced to provide for themselves (Dohm, *Emancipation* 54). Similarly, Morgenstern refers to such a way of thinking as the "Geschlechtsdespotismus" and the "Willkür des Mannes" (21).

3.5 The Female Body in the Private Realm

In the introduction to this chapter, I demonstrated that the perception of specific gender characteristics in conjunction with class differences had significant consequences for spatial politics. In her article "Die weibliche Ehre," Raschke states that the division between the private and the public space is simultaneously a gender division: "'Die Frau gehört ins Haus!' Nur die von vier Wänden eingeschlossene Welt soll die ihre sein; sie soll weder sehen noch wissen, was

173 Dohm does not identify him.

außerhalb dieses engbegrenzten Raumes geschieht. [...] Der Mann gehört in die Welt. Die Höhen und Tiefen des Menschenlebens sind ihm bekannt" ("Die weibliche Ehre" 250). She points out that the public space, including the privilege of education, was a male domain from which women were generally excluded. According to this logic, there was no reason for a middle-class woman to leave the private realm, since her existence was defined in terms of reproduction and her husband's pleasure. Therefore, a woman's freedom of movement was limited to the private space and her transgression into the public realm was strictly controlled by moral standards, to which she had no choice but to conform, as well as by law enforcement agencies such as the *Sittenpolizei*. As if to prove the accuracy of Raschke's claims, Waldeyer indicated that a woman has the greatest appeal for men when she is confined to the private realm: "[D]ie Frau bleibe [...] in demjenigen Kreise, in welchem sie ihre natürliche Kraft und Entwicklungsfähigkeit besitzt. Sie wird dann dem Manne begehrenswerth erscheinen, wie der in seiner Sphäre tüchtige Mann dem Weibe" (43).

Since the middle-class woman was expected to confine herself primarily to the private realm, it is not surprising that female knowledge was defined as "nichts anderes als Küchen- und Wäscheweisheit" (Beruna 13). Implied in the separation of space into male and female zones is simultaneously a division of knowledge along gender lines. While any type of knowledge was easily available to middle-class men, women had only limited access to it. These men could experience life as they pleased, had access to education, and had no knowledge boundaries imposed on them. Women's knowledge, on the other hand, was, in general, restricted due to their "Verbannung in die Küche" (Beruna 40) and to a large extent mediated by men. According to Mazón, it was even deemed inappropriate "for young women to read daily newspapers with their political contents" (16-17). It becomes evident that a woman's ideal confinement to the private space simultaneously created epistemological boundaries.[174]

The exclusion of middle-class women from the public space was based on the popular conviction that women were biologically not predisposed to process a large number of external stimuli. Only a confinement to the private space made it possible for women to avoid over-stimulation of their nervous system that could potentially lead to a serious mental disorder.[175] Hence, medical guidance for women of the time consisted mainly of advising them to stay at home and rest. Charlotte Perkins Gilman demonstrated the devastating consequences such a

174 While discussing the notion of *Wissenschaft* in the context of a male student's participation in the intellectual life of the university, Mazón agues that "*Wissenschaft* was gendered on two levels. First, the cultivation of an educated, independent judgment [...] was a process reserved almost exclusively for men. Second, the internalizing of knowledge [...] rested in masculine images of power and appropriation" (37).

175 The connection between exclusion of women from the public space and the nineteenth-century conviction that women were biologically not predisposed to process a large number of external stimuli was suggested by Professor Jennifer Terry in one of our conversations.

"therapy" had for women in her well-known story *The Yellow Wallpaper* (1892). In the German context, Dohm calls attention to the fact that it is precisely the confinement to the private realm with its prison-like qualities that makes women neurotic. She argues that it is the private, not the public space, in which women tend to lose control over their emotions. She claims that the most dramatic tragedies of female existence (such as physical abuse) take place at home. However, contrary to the evidence of these tragedies as reported by daily newspapers, many of which result in homicide ("Gattenmord") (Dohm, *Emancipation* 75), society still feels more comfortable if the middle-class woman's existence is restricted to the private realm. Dohm perceives a collective irrational fear of a middle-class woman leaving the private realm: "So schreckliche Dinge sind zu befürchten, wenn die Frauen außerhalb des Hauses ins volle Menschenleben greifen wollen; nicht aber ist zu befürchten, daß innerhalb der vier Wände ihr Gefühl jemals mit dem Verstande in Collision gerathe" (*Emancipation* 74).

Many activists saw bourgeois marriage as an institution that perpetuated female subjugation and confined women to the private realm. Hainisch, for instance, traces the history of women's oppression and sees its foundation in the marriage practices of the pre-Christian Germans to which she refers to as "die erste und entscheidende Ursache der Frauenerniedrigung" (*Seherinnen* 6). Similarly, Mayreder critiques the institution of marriage for its power to strip woman of her personality ("Die schöne Weiblichkeit" 121-122). Stolle compares marriage to prison (76) and indicates that a woman is entirely powerless and always dependent on her husband within this institution. He, in turn, acquires "property rights" to his wife:

> Wenn vor dem Standesbeamten die üblichen Formalitäten erfüllt sind, dann ist das Zusammenleben vor den Augen der Welt ein ehrenvolles, und wie viel Schmach und Schande kann oft dies vom Gesetz geheiligte Zusammenleben einem Weibe bringen! Wenn der Mann ein Trunkenbold ist oder ein ausschweifender Wüstling, der jedes höhere, reine, edle Empfinden einer Frau mit Füßen tritt, er aber unumschränkte Macht über das ihm gehörende Weib hat, kann man sich eine größere Entehrung, eine tiefere Schmach vorstellen, als einem solchen entarteten Mann sich willenlos hingeben zu müssen? (Stolle 51-52)

Stolle's book with its self-explanatory title, *Sklavenketten der Frauen*, does not explicitly address the question of medical education for women. Unlike other intellectuals and activists discussed thus far, Stolle does not demand women's admission to universities. On the contrary, she argues that a woman's entrance into the professional world is not supported by biological factors and would necessarily cause degeneration of the following generations (85). In other words, she does not propose professional emancipation as a solution of the "Woman Question."

However, Stolle's book clearly demonstrates the politics of gendered knowledge and the restrictions imposed on women within the private realm. Hence, the analysis of her text permits a more nuanced representation of certain women's perspectives on femininity.

Stolle extensively addresses the problem of women's subjugation in the private realm, the cause of which she sees in the male perception of women as one-dimensional sexual beings. According to Stolle, sexual relations between men and women are the major issue to be addressed by the women's movement. She contends: "So lange die Auffassung der Männer über die Frauen als Geschlechtswesen keine andere geworden, ist der Frauenbewegung von Anfang an der richtige Boden genommen" (Stolle 9). Consequently, she is an outspoken advocate of equal rights in the realm of sexuality. In this context, Stolle investigates three main issues: prostitution, gender-specific moral standards, and marriage. I focus on her claims pertaining to the confinement of middle-class women to the private realm. Particularly, I explore the regulations imposed on women by marriage and the restrictions placed on women's knowledge regarding their bodies and sexuality.

The correlation between the spatial and epistemological politics imposed on the female body was addressed by many early feminists. Because the exclusion of women from the public space was simultaneously an exclusion from knowledge about the world and about their own bodies, the connection between a woman's sexual knowledge and the resistance to the admission of women to medical schools is evident. As I have suggested above, the resistance to the admission of women to medical schools has one of its roots in the anxiety about women's transgression of spatial and epistemological boundaries. Upon entering medical schools, women would be included in the realm of knowledge about gendered bodies. Consequently, as physicians, they would participate in the production and distribution of medical knowledge.[176]

It is difficult to claim with certainty how much middle-class women knew about sexuality and bodily functions before or even after marriage. Many female activists of the nineteenth century indicated that this knowledge was, indeed, very limited. They pointed out that the upbringing of middle-class girls made inquiries into the subject almost impossible; sexuality was a subject bourgeois women did not address. Upon marriage, women were confronted with their sexuality.[177] Many texts indicate that such a confrontation could be quite traumatic. Stolle states: "Entsetzlich ist es, wenn sich die satte, abgelebte Sinnlichkeit mit der unentweihten Keuschheit vermählt, und es ist nur richtig und notwendig, daß die Mädchen nicht wie bisher so in der Dummheit erhalten bleiben. Die Macht darf nicht in einer Hand liegen, dann muß Sklaventum entstehen" (Stolle 84). Binder represents a similar point of view: "Wie unwissend und dadurch zugleich unbeschützt läßt man alljährlich tausende von jungen Mädchen in die Fremde gehen, [...] wie

176 See footnote 154.

177 Thorson discusses representation of this problem in a novel by Grete Meisel-Hess, *Fanny Roth*, 219-223.

unwissend überantwortet man die junge Frau dem oft keineswegs vernünftigen Gatten" (66). Another female activist, the previously mentioned Dr. H. Paul comments extensively on women's ignorance regarding sexual knowledge as perpetuated by the upbringing and moral standards of the middle class: "Jeder Einblick in ihre [der Frau] eigene Natur ist ihr verwehrt. *Sie darf nichts über sich selbst wissen!* [...] das wäre im höchsten Grade unweiblich. Ihr eigener Körper muß ihr ein Geheimnis, ein Rätsel bleiben!" (21). Although Paul admits that it might seem unbelievable, she claims that: "Es gibt junge Frauen, die eine Stunde vor ihrer Entbindung noch nicht wissen, auf welche Weise ein Kind geboren wird" (22). Such a claim is supported by the feminist scholar Londa Schiebinger. Although Schiebinger refers to the lack of knowledge of contraception, she also implies that in the nineteenth century, women's sexual knowledge was almost non-existent:

> Within Europe the decline of midwifery undermined traditional knowledge of contraception—knowledge that had typically passed along women's networks from mother to daughter, midwife to neighbor. As a result, European women of the nineteenth century had more children than their grandmothers did and understood less about their own bodies. (110)

Schiebinger argues that the lack of female-mediated sexual knowledge had negative consequences for women's understanding of their own bodies. She also claims that prior to the nineteenth century, women had access to "experts in women's health who were neither academic physicians nor barber-surgeons" (Schiebinger 110). However, this situation changed when "[f]emale practitioners were not accepted as co-professionals in the nineteenth century, but were excluded from medical schools. As a result women became more and more dependent on university-trained physicians for their care" (Schiebinger 110). Consequently, the knowledge of the female body was mediated exclusively by men. Hence, we can understand the demand for the admission of women to medical schools also as an attempt to empower women by providing them with female-mediated professional knowledge about their own bodies.[178]

Paul argues that a middle-class woman's lack of knowledge about sexuality is perpetuated and driven by male interests:

> Dem Manne ist die Unwissenheit seiner Frau recht, denn er liebt es nicht, daß die Frau so klug sei, als er selbst, es wäre manchem vielleicht unangenehm. Er kommt sich groß vor als der allein Gebende und die Frau hat zufrieden zu sein, mit dem was er ihr gibt. Manche junge Frauen haben im Anfange ihrer Ehe das Unglaublichste von perversen Männern erduldet [...] weil sie glaubten, "es gehöre sich

178 The question of women's knowledge will be addressed in Chapter Four.

> so." [...] Die Männer wollen zudem eine unwissende Frau, weil es ihnen behagt, sie in jeder Beziehung abhängig zu wissen. Ein Weib, das ganz genau weiß, was es vom Manne zu erfordern und zu erwarten hat, würde ihm unbequem sein [...]. (22-23)

Although Paul, like Stolle, does not explicitly discuss the issue of female medical doctors, her arguments gain an additional dimension in the context of the debate about admission of women to medical schools. Many progressive writers emphasized not only the importance of women having access to female doctors, but also the necessity of hiring female doctors in schools for girls. Girls would learn about their bodies and sexuality from women competent to mediate such knowledge. The medical profession would make this special kind of knowledge, insight into the mysteries of the human body, accessible to women.

As noted in Chapter One, in the case of bourgeois women, the notion of virginity encompassed much more than just a purely physical dimension. In addition, it implied lack of exposure to the knowledge about sexuality and limited presence in the public space. Dohm points out that as a consequence of such an understanding of virginity, "zarte Unwissenheit" and "Seelen-Unberührtheit" (*Emancipation* 130) developed as markers of moral standards applied to young women. She stipulates further that these features are cultivated by men "mehr aus ästhetischen und sinnlichen, als aus sittlichen Motiven" (*Emancipation* 130). At the same time, she complains that "die Unkenntnis der physischen Vorgänge für heilig gilt und als Schutz der weiblichen Tugend gepriesen wird" (*Emancipation* 131). She also rejects the notion of "Befleckung der Frauenseele durch das Studium" (Dohm, *Emancipation* 130). Similarily, Marie Borostyani points out that the alleged connection between medical education of women and their symbolic loss of virginity is created by the "Eitelkeit der Männer": "Viele auch wollen die Frauen von diesem oder jenem Zweige des Wissens ferne halten, weil sie ihn nicht für anständig halten für sie. Es gibt jedoch keine Wissenschaft, welche nicht an und für sich anständig wäre und welche die Keuschheit, Anständigkeit und Würde der Frau verletzen könnte [...]" (76).

In order to sustain the notion of virginity encompassing body, knowledge, and confinement in the private sphere, the development of young women is artificially suppressed. As Mayreder notes: "Die Methode der weiblichen Erziehung ist darauf gerichtet, einen selbständigen Entwicklungsprozess hintanzuhalten; sie ist eine Methode der Unterdrückung, der Einschüchterung, der künstlichen Wachsthumsverhinderung" ("Die schöne Weiblichkeit" 122). Paul refers to this process as a mutilation of the female soul: "[...] Seele wird gleichsam kastriert, damit der Körper 'intakt' bleibt" (21).

3.6 The Public Space of the University

As demonstrated above, bourgeois women's exclusion from the public realm was based on its sexualization and on gender-specific assignment of space. Additionally, middle-class moral standards restricted women's movement. Griselda Pollock notes that the public space was perceived as potentially dangerous for middle-class women:

> For bourgeois women, mingling with crowds of mixed social composition was not only frightening because it became increasingly unfamiliar, but because it was morally dangerous. It had been argued that to maintain one's respectability, closely identified with femininity, meant not exposing oneself in public. The public space was officially the realm of and for men; for women to enter it entailed unforeseen risks. (Pollock 69)[179]

This passage suggests a connection between the sexualization of the public space and its designation as dangerous for women. A story told by Stolle demonstrates the accuracy of this observation. It concerns a young woman she personally knew who made her living by taking on sewing work and doing it at home. Offered a much better job as a saleswoman, she refused to accept it. Asked why, she replied: "Ach, da giebt es zu viel Gefahren für ein junges Mädchen, und ich möchte doch nicht gern schlecht werden. In solchem Handschuhgeschäft müssen die Verkäuferinnen freundlich zu den kaufenden Herren sein und auf Verlangen des Abends mit ihnen ausgehen, sonst verliert sich die Kundschaft" (Stolle 63). The story indicates that a woman's presence in the public space implies her sexual availability. Pollock also notes in a different context that certain "territories of the bourgeois city [...] became the sites for the negotiation of gendered class identities and class gender positions" (70). I propose that at the end of the nineteenth century, the public space of the university became the site for the negotiation of a new female identity: the educated, confident, and independent middle-class woman, a woman who can "scharf denken," "schnell handeln," and "energisch zugreifen" (Schirmacher, "Die akademische Frau" 28). The struggle over the admission of women to medical schools and universities in Austria and Germany demonstrates the intricacy of the process in which new gender identities are negotiated.

Warning against women's entrance to the university, the opponents usually evoke two different scenarios. The first typically involves a number of variations on the "Entweiblichung des Weibes" (Irma von Troll-Borostyáni, "Etwas über Weiblichkeit" 811). In this case, as discussed above, woman undergoes a transformation into a "Mannweib," beast, sexually perverted individual, or a cold-blooded sadist to name only a few of these. Dohm emphasizes such a perception of female students:

179 Also qtd. in Parons 59.

> Und diese unberechenbaren Weiber, diese Sphinxe – nein, diese Medusen der Wissenschaft, vor denen alle Idealität erstarrt, sobald sie auf der Schwelle der Universität erscheinen! Daheim aber tritt (wie es nach den herkömmlichen Phrasen heißt) Idealität, Poesie und alles Schöne und Herrliche mit ihnen über die Schwelle des Hauses! (*Emancipation* 135)

The second scenario creates an entirely different picture of female students. They are targets of advances or victims of sexual assaults undertaken by their male peers. What is striking in both cases is the focus on female sexuality and its exaggerated proportions. In the first situation (excluding "Mannweib"), the female student becomes an aggressive sexual predator. In the second setting, she is turned into a passive victim of male sexual drives.

The second scenario is clearly evoked in Bischoff's writings. As Dohm points out, according to him, one of the obstacles preventing women from entering medical schools is the rudeness and brutality of male students ("Rohheit der Studenten") (*Emancipation* 132). Bischoff argues that in the university space, women would be continuously exposed to sexual harassment due to the natural sexual drive of all men including male students:

> [S]o unterliegt es doch keinem Zweifel, daß derselbe [der weibliche Theil der Zuhörerschaft] beständigen Angriffen von Seiten des männlichen Theiles ausgesetzt sein wird; [...] Die Studentinnen [...] werden entweder dem fortwährenden Andrange von Seiten der männlichen Zuhörerschaft erliegen, oder wenn sie ihm Widerstand leisten, so wird die unausbleibliche Folge Anfeindnungen, Beleidigungen, Spott, Streitig-keiten der Studenten untereinander u.s.w. sein. (Bischoff 40)[180]

The ideological basis of such claims is apparent. The endangerment is depicted as both inevitable and natural, without any questioning of woman's status as a sexual object in the social/male consciousness. The solution grants men greater freedom by restricting female autonomy, and not only in the sexual realm. As indicated by Bischoff's statement, men are not forced to take control of their sexual drive; instead women have to avoid male harassment by renouncing the public space.

In contrast, Dohm insists on protecting women by restricting male—not female—freedom:

> Betragen die Studenten sich pöbelhaft gegen Damen, so jage man sie von der Universität weg *(wegen mißliebiger politischer Äußerungen*

180 Also qtd. in Dohm, *Emancipation* 132.

hat man früher dasselbe gethan), oder man sperre sie, je nach dem Maß ihrer Rohheit, auf längere oder kürzere Zeit ins Karzer (*Emancipation* 134; emphasis added).

Dohm indicates that gender politics is an ideology and can be imposed by the university authorities. The law reinforces traditional gender relations by withholding certain rights from women, for example, access to education, the right to be gainfully employed, and the right to vote. At the same time, Dohm acknowledges that legal regulations can be changed and that women can influence laws in their struggle for education. Of course, many feminists chose this path by petitioning legal authorities.

The ideological struggle over the contested space of the university is illustrated by the following incident. A feminist journal *Dokumente der Frauen* reported, in its April 1, 1899 issue, the protest of male students against women's participation in clinical courses at the university in Halle ("Notizen" 42).[181] However, in this case, the university authorities proved to be much more open-minded than the students: "[...] das Decanat der medicinischen Fakultät in Halle, die einzig kompetente Instanz in dieser Frage, zieh diese sonderbaren Idealisten öffentlich der Lüge, erklärte ihre Beschwerde für vollkommen grundlos und bedauerte die Animosität gegen die weiblichen Studierenden, [...]" ("Notizen" 42). This incident demonstrates that in some cases authorities decided to reinforce non-traditional gender relations by using legislative and executive prerogatives. The professors in Halle also deemed the protest to be a manifestation of "egoistischen Sonderinteressen" ("Notizen" 42) that, they argued, should be excluded from scientific pursuit. The reaction of the university authorities and professors in this case represents one of the first successes of the women's movement regarding the negotiation of new gender identities.

181 See also Bandhauer-Schöffmann 66; Mazón 125-126.

4 The Woman's Reproductive Body and Scientific Production of Knowledge

Our bodies, as well as the world we live in, are certainly made of materials. And we often use scientific investigation to understand the nature of those materials. But such scientific investigation involves a process of knowledge construction.

Anne Fausto-Sterling[182]

There is no such thing as apolitical science.

Anne Fausto-Sterling[183]

The biology of sexual difference is embedded in other cultural programs.

Thomas Laqueur[184]

4.1 Introduction: Conflicting Views on Female Reproductive Physiology

Proponents of higher education for women who responded to specific texts written by medical doctors intervened in the medical discourse in order to show that what was supposed to be objective scientific knowledge was manipulated to fit a specific ideological agenda. This intervention was important for two reasons. First, many physicians and scientists claimed to speak from the position of medical authority about the female bodily experience and assumed the universality of their claims. Critics responding to these pamphlets, both men and women, demonstrated that women actually could experience their bodies differently than described by medical doctors. Simultaneously, they negated the accuracy of some of the medical observations, particularly those that were believed to make higher education for women impossible. Second, since the pamphlets written by opponents of medical education for women were directed to a wide audience and not exclusively to the medical community, it was important to challenge their claims publicly and to correct or modify their statements as well as to produce and disseminate an alternative interpretation of biological data and processes.

As noted in the preceding chapters, popular medical texts that discussed the issue of "female nature" in the context of academic education portrayed men and women as two different and incompatible species and focused on the differences between the sexes. The authors primarily emphasized the limitations imposed on women by their bodies and physiological functions. During the last decade of the nineteenth century, scientists and physicians who opposed women's entrance into

182 *Sexing the Body* 28.
183 *Myths of Gender* 207.
184 *Making Sex. Body and Gender from the Greeks to Freud* 19.

the world of academic education attempted to bring to public attention what they believed to be the incapacitating effects of the female reproductive physiology. From their perspective, the female body was an imperfect version of the male body in a state of permanent impairment[185] manifested through and symbolized by menstruation. Women could not overcome the limitations imposed by their anatomy and especially by their reproductive physiological functions. Men, on the other hand, were not limited by their bodies and many physicians argued that male bodily functions did not impose any restrictions on men's lives. The fusion of the physical, intellectual, spiritual, and moral dimensions in women corresponded to a separation of these faculties in men. While the male's cognitive ability allowed him to transcend the physical principle by participating in the spiritual and intellectual realm, the female was bound by and limited to the physical aspects of her body. Thus, opponents of women's education focused entirely on the boundaries of the female body in their discussion of gender limitations. Many progressive intellectuals of the nineteenth century, on the contrary, reached beyond these boundaries in an attempt to prove that the female sex too can be transcended.

Since bourgeois women, according to the established social order, did not have any purpose of existence beyond serving their husbands and children, we can understand the female body as traditionally regulated through three closely connected categories: physical attraction, male pleasure, and reproductive sexuality. Texts opposing higher education for women evoke these categories as the main parameters for the bourgeois woman's existence. Since academic education was unquestionably beyond these categories, it was conventionally not a desirable element in bourgeois women's life. On the contrary, as demonstrated in the preceding chapter, it was even regarded as a potential threat to the reproductive functions and aesthetics of the female body.

While most of the male medical theorists hold onto a formula that equates women with their bodies, many progressive individuals attempt to destabilize this cultural construction of femininity and move beyond the body itself. By so doing, they assert the subjectivity of the female body. In addition, many women provide different interpretations of their bodily reproductive functions. Unlike most of the male scientists, these women do not see menstruation, pregnancy, and childbearing and rearing as disruptive or otherwise incapacitating processes in their lives. Instead, they provide a new interpretation of these processes and their impact on a woman's life. However, although these women attempt to redefine the notion of femininity based on their own understanding of their bodies, they are conditioned, nonetheless, by the ideological frameworks and institutional practices of the time.

The point of departure for this chapter is a text by Max Runge, *Das Weib in seiner geschlechtlichen Eigenart*, and the responses it generated. Runge was a professor of gynecology and obstetrics at the Georg-August-University in Göttingen between 1888 and 1909. His two pamphlets, *Das Weib in seiner geschlechtlichen*

185 See footnote 156.

Eigenart (1896) and *Männliche und weibliche Frauenheilkunde* (1899), defended the position that women were neither suited for academic pursuits nor needed as physicians. Both pamphlets were based on lectures at the Georg-August-University. They drew substantial attention and numerous critical reviews and not only in the feminist press. Public responses to Runge's texts, which significantly exceeded reactions to other earlier misogynist writings, permit the conclusion that the women's cause was becoming increasingly more popular and had gained a number of supporters. My analysis encompasses the most detailed and elaborate reactions to Runge's *Das Weib in seiner geschlechtlichen Eigenart*: Marie Brühl's *Die Natur der Frau und Herr Professor Runge*, Frieda Freiin von Bülow's "Das Weib in seiner Geschlechtsindividualiät," Fritz Brupbacher's *Geburtshelfer Runge und die Frauen-Emanzipation,* Heinrich Meyer's "Professor Runge und die Frauen," and Hedwig Dohm's "Die Ritter der *mater dolorosa*."

4.2 Max Runge's *Das Weib in seiner geschlechtlichen Eigenart*

Runge's theories of female inferiority move away from the analysis of the brain's capacity and structure to an examination of female reproductive organs and their functions. His focus on reproductive organs is understandable due to Runge's medical specialization. However, it is also connected to a more general development in the medical field, specifically the rise of gynecology as a new scientific discipline during the course of the nineteenth century.[186] Schmersahl points out that "[d]ie Gynäkologie, die bis zum 19. Jahrhundert teils in chirurgischen, teils in innermedizinischen, teils in geburtshilferischen Händen gelegen hatte, begann sich etwa ab 1860 als eigenständige medizinische Spezialdisziplin herauszubilden" (196).[187] The first German gynecological textbook, written by Carl Gustav Carus and published in 1820, derived woman's position in society, her general physiological and psychological health (or lack thereof), her cognitive abilities, as well as her personality and character from her sexuality (Schmersahl 192). Further gynecological research confirmed Carus' findings and, as Schmersahl puts it, "die Gynäkologen der zweiten Hälfte des 19. Jahrhunderts [waren sich] darüber [einig], daß die Geschlechtsfunktionen im engeren oder weiteren Sinne das Sein der Frauen determinierten" (193). Schmersahl argues that, by claiming the alleged close connection between woman's reproductive physiology and her psyche, gynecologists were able "das Denken und Fühlen von Frauen sowie deren soziales Verhalten aus klinischer Sicht zu kontrollieren" (311). By connecting all areas of woman's life, directly or indirectly, to her sexuality, gynecologists could claim to be the ultimate experts on anything concerning women[188] and they did stake this

186 See Schmersahl 190-212.

187 See also Schmersahl's footnote 22 (196).

188 Schmersahl refers to "die Entwicklung der Gynäkologie im 19. Jahrhundert, in dem sich Frauenärzte zu Fachmännern für 'Frauenfragen' aufschwangen" (190). See also Schmersahl 310.

claim, especially to oppose women's emancipation, in general, and access to higher education, in particular (Schmersahl 190; 194-95; 310-12).

Runge followed in his predecessors' footsteps by arguing that woman's nature derives from her sexual specificity and most female qualities can be explained as being connected to a woman's reproductive functions. This claim is already suggested by the title of Runge's pamphlet, which depicts a woman's sexuality as inferior and deviant if measured against "the norm" that is male. Since all differences between men and women derive from their sexual dissimilarities, men and women are consequently diametrically opposed to and incompatible with each other. Therefore, according to Runge, there is no basis for the social equality of both genders and such is not desirable.

Runge argues that the "Studium der geschlechtlichen Eigenart des Weibes" (*Eigenart* VI) should constitute the basis for political decisions about the role, rights, and privileges of women in society. Consequently, he understands gynecology as the science of woman, able to explain all aspects of female existence, interpret female nature, and find solutions for the "Woman Question." By the same token, a gynecologist is best suited to analyze the nature, abilities, and the role of women in society. Already at the very beginning of his text, Runge attempts to establish his authority as the expert in all questions pertaining to women due to his belief that the female physiology and reproductive functions determine all aspects of a woman's life.

Accordingly, Runge polarizes male and female existence into the realm of intellect and the realm of reproduction. He quotes the writer Nikolaus Lenau to make this division explicit: "Was für den Mann Erkenntniskraft, ist für das Weib die Mutterschaft" (Runge, *Eigenart* 11). Lenau refers to the established binary oppositions between man/brain/intellect and woman/uterus/physicality. The focus on female physiological functions allows Runge to see women as limited entirely to the physical dimension of their bodies and their reproductive functions. He emphasizes that women's bodies are subjected to eternal rules of nature from which they cannot deviate. Since female lives are centered around and regulated by reproductive functions, and since, according to Runge, female health depends on the fulfillment of reproductive functions, women are dependent on men. He calls this dependency "Naturnotwendigkeit" and argues that women who do not fulfill their reproductive functions degenerate into hysterics (Runge, *Eigenart* 12). Hence, the fulfillment of the reproductive functions is essential for sustaining female health. Only through the processes of pregnancy and childbearing can a woman achieve her full potential. Women who do not become mothers deteriorate physically because they do not comply with the rules of nature. Men, on the other hand, are self-sufficient and independent. They are not limited by their physiology and are biologically not determined to the same degree as women. Unlike women, they are multidimensional beings, easily able to transcend bodily boundaries through their intellect. Their role is to explore the world, support and protect the family while the reproductive functions play only a marginal role in their lives. While a woman's "profession" is to give birth and rear children, a man's life encompasses remuneration and work in the public space. Runge refers to reproduction as "Berufstätigkeit des Weibes" (*Eigenart* 6) and "der natürliche *Beruf des Weibes*" (*Eigenart* 9). By regularly fulfilling their reproductive functions, women utilize and develop the potential of their nature. By pursuing higher education, women not only deflect their energy from procreation but also jeopardize their reproductive sexuality.

Runge devotes a large part of his pamphlet to a discussion of menstruation, pregnancy, and birth because he sees women through the prism of these processes. He defines menstruation as "reizbare Schwäche" (*Eigenart* 3), by which women's efficiency and productivity in all areas of life is dramatically reduced. It is precisely during these times that women require extensive care and have to renounce all other activities. According to Runge, menstruation is a main source of a woman's physical and mental weakness and has negative effects on her potential achievements. This negative impact of menstruation is doubled in the case of female participation in higher education because the general weakness caused by menstruation increases if accompanied by intellectual work (Runge, *Eigenart* 5). In other words, any intellectual pursuit advances the physical weakness caused by the physiological processes. Women who work intellectually are not able to fulfill their reproductive function properly and suffer significant impairments that other women do not. Hence, intellectual work and child bearing are mutually exclusive (Runge, *Eigenart* 38). Therefore, the pursuit of intellectual work by women is seen as a female whim, a personal egotism that leads to degeneration (Runge, *Eigenart* 38).

Female physiology and biological factors sabotage women's demands for equality. The processes of pregnancy, giving birth, and nurturing are more demanding than menstruation and require more physical and mental energy, further diminishing a woman's productivity (Runge, *Eigenart* 5). Due to these processes, women suffer physical pain and are exposed to potential health challenges that, naturally, do not affect men. Runge describes, for example, giving birth as "ein Vorgang mit höchst mangelhaften und unvollkommenen Einrichtungen" (*Eigenart* 6-7) because it can lead to a number of complications. Additionally, women suffer from a "Geburtswunde" (*Eigenart* 7) that, according to Runge, impacts female health for many years. Therefore Runge contends that a woman's physical constitution is less perfect than a man's: "Die Organisation des Weibes für seinen Beruf ist [...] zweifellos eine unvollkommenere, als die des Mannes für den seinigen" (*Eigenart* 7). It is due to this imperfection that women are much more likely than men to be susceptible to sexually transmitted diseases and also tend to develop any type of sickness to a much higher degree and severity than men. This susceptibility to illness increases if any intellectual work is done. Physical and mental weakness caused by reproductive processes forces women to forgo all other activities. Consequently, Runge equates female existence with pain and renunciation. Woman, then, emerges as a flawed version of the human being.

Although Runge seems to classify women in terms of the "proper" functioning of the reproductive organs, as signified by menstruation and pregnancy, he also perceives female sexuality as a sign of women's inferiority in relation to men. On a physical level, menstruation is described in terms of sickness and, one could conclude, it is almost portrayed as an anomaly that signifies a deficient development of a human being. On a metaphorical level, it is regarded as a symbol of this very imperfection. Hence, physical imperfection is considered to be inherent in the female body. In other words, the physical imperfection constitutes the basis of a perfectly functioning female body. Menstruation is both a manifestation and a symbol of this imperfection or degeneration. Similarly, Dr. Placzek, a Berlin physician, argues that "[d]as Weib ist nur in Intervallen eines beständigen Krankseins gesund" (qtd. in Dohm, "Die Ritter" 35).[189] The core of this sickness is the female sex; in other words, womanhood itself is the woman's sickness.[190] Although the prominent sexologist Havelock Ellis argued that one cannot denote a bodily function as a sickness if half of all human beings are subject to it (Tichy, "Die geschlechtliche Un-Ordnung" 34), the popular belief coincided with Runge's. The majority of the opponents of academic education for women cited pregnancy and menstruation along with the absence of a "properly" functioning brain as the biggest obstacle for the potential female students.

Runge contends that the female nature and character derive from a woman's sexual organs. Since the female reproductive organs are believed to be less perfect than those of men, the female character that is derived from these organs is flawed. In fact, Runge believes that due to the shame women experience because of the visible manifestation of their sexuality such as menstruation and pregnancy, they developed a tendency to hide such manifestations and as a result, they also acquired a predisposition to cheating and lying in general. Thus, women are doomed to despise truth and honesty to a much higher degree than men (Runge, *Eigenart* 21-22). According to Runge, each woman has "eine Neigung zur Täuschung und zum Trug" and is "weniger wahrheitsliebend [...] als der Mann" (*Eigenart* 21-22). An inclination to devote attention to appearance and a craving for admiration ("Putz," "Gefallsucht") (Runge, *Eigenart* 25) constitute the second set of typically female characteristics. Runge argues that because women need men in order to fulfill their purpose in life and to maintain physical and mental health, they attempt to attract men by any means.[191] In contrast, the main male character trait derived from his sexuality is brutality. According to Runge it is impossible to eliminate male physical or sexual brutality because it is inherent. Consequently, moral and sexual rules of conduct were created in order to protect women from male brutality. These morals and customs, including the restriction of

189 See also Schmersahl 307.

190 See footnote 156.

191 This statement is reminiscent of the misogynistic article by Wittels analyzed in Chapter Three.

women to the private sphere, are necessary as "heilsame Schranken" (Runge, *Eigenart* 29) to protect women.[192]

4.3 The Question of Knowledge Production

Runge participates in the production and dissemination of knowledge that relegates female reproductive sexuality to the realm of destructive and irrational forces. Female reproductive sexuality is defined as an all-encompassing principle, "die dunkle Basis der Weibnatur" (Runge 17),[193] that leaves women prone to diseases, intellectually challenged, physically weak, morally questionable, and not able to undertake any other activity. The female body is not seen in itself as life-giving, but rather as defective matter, or, as Emily Martin puts it, "the 'raw material' from which the 'product' [baby] is extracted" (19).

The responses to Runge's pamphlet challenge the dominant medical practice as the authoritative and exclusive source of knowledge about women. Dohm identifies texts written by the orthodox opponents of higher education for women as symptomatic of the lack of ideological stability in relation to gender. Pamphlets such as Runge's *Das Weib in seiner geschlechtlichen Eigenart* attest to a destabilization of traditional gender models. The very fact that numerous attacks on educational demands were made by scientists and physicians as well as the orthodoxy of these attacks exemplify this ideological instability. In addition, Dohm contends that the arguments of the orthodox opponents of women's medical education such as Runge and Placzek are self-referential and dogmatic. These claims originate in a frame of mind that manipulates the evidence in order to prove that the particular view is universal. Likewise, Frieda von Bülow asserts in her response to Runge that his convictions are logically indefensible: "Wer seine Lehre mit Scheingründen und beliebig aufgegriffenen Nebensächlichkeiten unterstützt, erweckt den Verdacht, Etwas zu vertreten, das sich ernsthaft nicht vertheidigen lässt" ("Das Weib" 596).

In his critique of Runge's pamphlet, Fritz Brupbacher, a Swiss physician who supported women's demands for medical education, focuses on the question of scientific accuracy.[194] He asserts the manipulative intentions of many scientists:

> Es wird in der Wissenschaft wohl nicht weniger mit unreellen Mitteln gekämpft als vor den Schranken des Gerichts, und jeder wirklich

192 This reminds us of Bischoff's argument against women's participation in higher education discussed in Chapter Three.

193 Runge uses the phrase "die Dunkle Basis der Weibnatur" in a passage in which he summarizes Laura Marholm's opinions about women's emancipation. It is not clear whether he cites this expression or whether it is his own.

194 The question of scientific accuracy was brought up in relation to Albert's pamphlet discussed in Chapter Three. It is one of the main problems associated with Albert, Runge, and Möbius.

Wissenwollende thut am besten, gar nicht an das, was ihm gelehrt wird, zu glauben, sondern erst was die eigenen Sinne als existierend, der eigene kritische Intellekt als richtig erprobt, als wissenschaftliche Erfahrung zu acceptieren. [...] so lange [...] das Gewissen unserer Gelehrten ein so unsauberes ist, wird uns kaum ein anderer Weg offen bleiben. (Brupbacher 1)

Brupbacher equates science with an ideological battlefield on which the ends seem to justify the means and they are, therefore, questionable. He declares that critical thinking should not only be a necessary part of scientific education, but that it also is a more reliable source of knowledge than mediated scientific inquiry. For Brupbacher, Runge's theories are among those not to be trusted. He relegates Runge's pamphlet to the realm of "pseudo-wissenschaftlicher Thätigkeit" (Brupbacher 1) and demonstrates "eine wirkliche Fälschung der wissenschaftlichen Thatsachen zu Gunsten der Ansicht" (Brupbacher 2) on Runge's part. He also brings up Runge's assertions concerning menstruation as "oberflächliche Behauptung" (Brupbacher 3) and, referring to scientific literature ("in jedem Handbuch der Frauenkrankheiten," Brupbacher 2), argues that the two (Runge's theory and scientific literature of the time) are not entirely compatible. Further, Brupbacher posits, quoting Schröder,[195] that "die Einwirkungen der Menstruation auf den Gesamtorganismus sind noch sehr wenig genau studiert. *Ja die Angaben darüber widersprechen sich nicht selten direkt*" (Brupbacher 3).[196] He points out that there is not enough scientific evidence for Runge's assertions, even though Runge depicts these theories as if they were established facts. Brupbacher draws the following conclusion: "Es ist ein Leichtsinn oder dann eine Unwahrhaftigkeit sondergleichen, uns zuzumuten, Runge solche Dinge zu glauben, die sonst nirgends stehen und die wir selbst nie zu erfahren die Gelegenheit haben" (4).

Even though Runge's theories of female reproductive sexuality as both all encompassing and destructive to women themselves are very radical and not shared by all members of the medical community, the author is nonetheless engaged in the production of knowledge that disseminates a distorted view of female sexuality for ideological reasons. Although the influence of such pamphlets on political decision-making has already been explained in Chapter Two, I would like to reiterate the importance of this connection by quoting one of Runge's adversaries, Heinrich Meyer, who emphasized the negative effects that Runge's speeches and pamphlets had produced: "[D]ie Meinung […] eines einflußreichen Professors an einer Universität [ist] etwas anderes als die Meinung eines beliebigen Privatmannes: sie zieht praktische Folgen nach sich [...]. Deshalb können wenigstens die interessierten Kreise an einer solchen offiziellen Kundgebung nicht achtlos vorübergehen" (711).

195 Brupbacher does not identify Schröder.

196 Brupbacher does not specify whether the emphasis is his or Schröder's.

In addition to their influence on political decision-making, these pamphlets had a significant impact on the general audience to which they were directed as well (Digby 208).[197] I suggest that the responses to Runge's pamphlet endeavor to correct the distorted view regarding female sexuality and reproductive functions in an attempt, at least, to counterbalance its negative impact on women's lives and on political decision-making. It is important to note that individuals who intervene in the production of knowledge about the female body often point out that physicians and scientists such as Runge and Placzek merely repeat the stereotypical views of gender differences that were neither groundbreaking nor true: "Alles, was Runge da sagt, sind Gemeinplätze, denen man so und so manchmal gegenteilige Beispiele entgegenhalten kann" (Brupbacher 12). Heinrich Meyer advances a similar argument:

> Trotz mancher interessanten Belehrung, die ja die Schriften von Prof. Runge unzweifelhaft enthalten, – in der eigentlichen Hauptfrage werden immer die altgewohnten Argumente ins Treffen geführt, die trotz unermüdlicher Wiederholung noch immer nicht wahrer und geistreicher geworden sind, und auch dadurch, daß ein deutscher Professor sie ausspricht, nicht an Gewicht gewinnen. (710)

In addition, Brupbacher recognizes that knowledge about the female body is not universal, but rather dependent on a specific social context. Therefore he declares Runge to be incompetent to talk about the "Woman Question," especially because "er noch nie Gelegenheit hatte, eine grössere Anzahl von Frauen zu sehen, die unter ganz anderen Bedingungen aufgewachsen sind, als die normale deutsche Hausfrau" (Brupbacher 11).

The question of scientific credibility is further complicated when Runge emphasizes the intricacy involved in the separation of the objective scientific analysis of the female body from the sexual appeal it has to heterosexual men. Runge reduces women to objects of male scientific investigation, but, at the same time, he admits that it is very difficult for men "objektiv [...] das Weib zu analysieren" (*Eigenart* 1). The separation of the two spheres is further complicated by the reduction of a woman's existence to her sexuality and by the perception of her as nothing but an object of male desire. The object of scientific analysis and the object of sexual desire seem to blend together, thus creating an inseparable entity. The fusion of these two spheres has significant implications for Runge's claims; it undermines his position to speak as an "infallible authority" about women:

197 Digby investigates a similar situation in Britan. She emphasizes the fact that many of the medical theories were directed to a general audience: "no longer content with the specialist pages of medical journals, they promoted their views in popular journals that would find readership in middle-class households" (208).

> Wenn die Frauenbewegung die Tendenz hat, das Weib zum Vollmenschen [...] zu entwickeln, dann hat sie keinen hartnäckigeren Gegner zu bekämpfen, als die alte, festgewurzelte Ansicht, die im Weibe nur oder vorwiegend das Geschlechtswesen sieht. Wem aber läge diese Auffassung näher als dem Frauenarzt, der mit dem Weibe eben nur als Körper, und zwar zunächst mit seiner sexuellen Sphäre zu thun hat [...]. (Meyer 711)

Obviously, the gynecologists' knowledge is restricted to the physicality and reproductive organs. Dohm, however, points out that they define themselves as specialists in all matters concerning women. Both Runge and Placzek "begnügen sich aber nicht, über die Physis der Frau ihr Verdikt abzugeben. Sie ziehen vielmehr aus ihrer körperlichen Bildung die kühnsten Schlussfolgerungen auf ihre geistige Beschaffenheit" (Dohm, "Die Ritter" 33). Therefore, according to Dohm, an objective analysis of female nature by a gynecologist is not possible.

4.4 Different Modes of Knowledge

The early feminists who responded to Runge provided a different perspective not only as to what constitutes femininity, but also with regard to the means by which this knowledge was produced. The position of power and authority allowed male scientists to regulate the female body by imposing certain modes of interpretation on women regarding the female bodily experience, they argued. However, in this case, the knowledge of the female body could only be external and theoretical, based on outside sources such as books, medical authority which was male biased, and in the best case on female-narrated experience.

Dohm complicates the question of knowledge about the female body by polarizing it as the realm of university education and the realm of personal experience:

> Es ist wahr, diese Herren [Runge und Placzek] haben den immensten Vorteil einer umfassenden Universitätsbildung vor mir voraus. Ich aber habe den Vorteil, *eine Frau* zu sein, also am eigenen Leibe die in Rede stehenden Vorgänge erfahren zu haben. Auch dürften die Mitteilungen kranker und gesunder Frauen an eine Geschlechtsgenossin und meine Erfahrungen und Beobachtungen an ihnen intimer und ausgiebiger sich erweisen, als die Auslassungen *nur* kranker Frauen an die Ärzte. ("Die Ritter" 33)

Dohm distinguishes here between two types of knowledge about women. One is produced by men in a university setting, at the laboratory, and in the physician's office. The other is the intuitive female knowledge of her own body. In addition, Dohm acknowledges that there are two ways in which this knowledge is disseminated and exchanged. In the first case, the basis of this knowledge is not so much the interaction between a male physician and a female patient as it is the interpretation of this interaction by the doctor. This implies an assumed superiority and imposition of the knowledge produced in a university setting on women, knowledge whose ownership is claimed by male doctors. In this instance, a woman does not have any agency over her own body and experience. In the second case, if women decide to talk to each other and share their experience, they reclaim the agency over their bodies because both of them mutually validate each other's personal knowledge.

Many supporters of medical education for women argued that a female physician would combine the positive aspects of both modes of knowledge, the theoretical and the empirical. Such knowledge would benefit all women because it would be more accurate and objective. Because, as I have previously noted, most proponents of women's medical education voiced the necessity to divide medical practices along gender lines, the argument needed only to be framed in terms of women and children. Female physicians were advocated for women and children, explicitly, and male doctors for men, implicitly. This division can be understood in two ways, on the one hand, as a tactical maneuver to establish women in the medical field and, on the other, as yet another reinforcement of the politics of sexual difference.[198]

Focusing on the female patient, Mathilde Weber perceives the blend of both modes of knowledge, the theoretical and the empirical, as necessary. The female patient would greatly benefit from physicians whose medical training incorporates "Behandlung und das *Studium unseres eigenen Körpers*" (Weber 32). She goes on to develop her argument as follows:

> Von wem erfahren denn die Ärzte unsere inneren gesundheitlichen Verhältnisse, nach welchen sie uns behandeln müssen? – durch *unsere* Auffassungen von unseren Schmerzen und Beschreibung unserer Empfindung. Warum sollte das eine Frau nicht ebenso an den anderen verstehen lernen, die dazu noch an sich selbst alles beobachten kann? (Weber 32)

Here, Weber stresses the question of the mediation of knowledge. According to her, female gynecologists would have a significant advantage over their male colleagues, because they have access to their own bodily experience in addition to

198 See also Hoesch 45. Mazón provides a similar argument. Many activists, she claims, such as Lange and Weber, emphasized "sexual difference" between men and women and instrumentalized it to argue for women's acces to education (75; 82). Weber and Lange also stressed the necessity "to give women access to selected professions [...]. By emphasizing only certain fields, Weber and Lange minimized misgivings about female competition and offered compelling arguments about the cultural and moral importance of women in these areas" (82). See also Mazón 106.

theoretical and mediated knowledge. Frieda von Bülow, too, deems the knowledge about women produced by physicians and professors in a hospital or at the university to be fragmented and insufficient: "Wir Frauen sind gewöhnt, von gelehrten Herren in einer Weise beurtheilt zu werden, die uns zeigt, daß trotz ihren theoretischen und praktischen Untersuchungen ihr Wissen und Begreifen auf diesem Gebiete gleich Null ist" ("Das Weib" 596). Bülow also contends that in order to gain a better understanding of the female body, the women's perspective and knowledge are crucial. Hence, she emphasizes the necessity to acknowledge the female voice.

Dohm, Bülow, and Brupbacher point to the regulatory aspect of the knowledge produced in a university setting. Without the theoretical knowledge about the female body created by male scientists and physicians, women experience their own bodies differently than if they had been exposed to it. In addition, women experience their bodies differently from the ways in which these men presume they do. For instance, Dohm contradicts Runge's assertions by evoking not only her own personal experiences, but also the experiences of many women in her family: "Wir Schwestern alle haben in jungen Jahren keine Ahnung davon gehabt, daß die Menstruation eine beachtenswerte Angelegenheit sei. *Niemand sagte es uns*" ("Die Ritter" 35; emphasis added). Women have *learned* to perceive their physiological functions such as menstruation according to the stigmatizing scientific view. Without scientific intervention, Dohm argues, menstruation is perceived by women just as one of many natural physiological functions.

In his analysis of menstruation and pregnancy, Runge describes this physiological process not as experienced by women, but as an experience imagined by men. Dohm shows that these two experiences are completely different. While a university-educated physician might have certain theoretical and clinical knowledge, he will not be able to liberate himself from his gender-determined outlook on these processes because they are alien to him and not accessible to the male through direct experience. Dohm, on the contrary, argues on the basis of her own experience: "Daß aber selbst ein hoher Grad von Übelbefinden während der Schwangerschaft mit geistiger oder körperlicher Arbeit sehr wohl vereinbar ist, *weiß ich wirklich besser, als irgend ein Arzt es wissen kann*" ("Die Ritter" 35; emphasis added). Therefore, she is able to claim authority over the interpretation of experiences and processes inherent to the female body. It is an authority that Runge obviously denies women. Dohm claims, for example, that contrary to Runge's opinion, intellectual work had helped her through physical suffering during a number of pregnancies:

> Während meiner fünf Schwangerschaften litt ich [...] ein Marthyrium [...]. So lange ich ruhelos und beschäftigungslos umherlief, war es am ärgsten. Da verfiel ich, um der Qual zu entgehen, darauf, spanische Verse [...] ins Deutsche zu übersetzen. Und das waren die einzigen erträglichen Stunden am Tage, wo ich in erregter geistiger

> Spannung, nach Worten und Reimen suchend, mich selbst und mein Leiden vergaß. ("Die Ritter" 35)

Thus, Dohm provides an alternative interpretation of the female experience of pregnancy. Similarly, she refers to her female family members, acquaintances, and friends who did not have to change their lives drastically while pregnant, which, again, contradicts the popular medical knowledge of the time (Dohm, "Die Ritter" 36). As a case in point she refers to her mother's experience:

> Meine Mutter hatte achtzehn Kinder. Als meine jüngsten Geschwister geboren wurden, war ich erwachsen. Und ich kann versichern, daß meine Mutter nie über irgend etwas klagte, daß sie vielmehr während der Schwangerschaften ihren riegoroßen [sic] Haushalt in derselben Rüstigkeit fortführte, wie zu jeder anderen Zeit. Von Nervosität, Kränkeleien – keine Spur! ("Die Ritter" 35)

Dohm concludes that "die krankhaften Erscheinungen bei vielen Frauen während der Schwangerschaft nicht auf einem Naturgesetz berufen, und daß sie bei rationeller und kraftvoller auferzogenen Geschlechtern der Zukunft zu den Ausnahmen gehören werden" ("Die Ritter" 36). These passages do not only illustrate the notion that scientific knowledge is dogmatic and not necessarily compatible with women's experiences, but they also hint at its capacity to create certain experiences that otherwise might not exist at all. Bülow provides a sarcastic reading of such a capacity to create new reality for women: "Von diesem Grade hoffnungslosen Jammers *hatten wir doch keine Ahnung!* Das ist zu viel! Krankheit, Schmerzen, Siechthum, wohin wir uns auch wenden!" (Bülow, "Das Weib" 597; emphasis added).

Besides distinguishing between theoretical knowledge and direct experience, many writers differentiate between knowledge about the healthy and the ill female body. Brupbacher, for instance, comments: "Man fragt sich wirklich [...] ob Runge überhaupt schon in der Lage war, eine gesunde Frau mit intellektueller Bildung zu sehen" (4). Similarly, Dohm claims that Runge, as a physician, interacts mainly with women in poor health. Therefore, he knows only a fragment of the female population: "Der Frauenarzt wird nur bei Geburten und bei Erkrankungen der weiblichen Sexualorgane zu Rate gezogen" ("Die Ritter" 33). She concludes that the male gynecologist is not competent to provide an expert opinion regarding female intellectual and spiritual capacities because he possesses only a one-sided and limited knowledge of women. Brühl takes this assertion even further arguing that this knowledge is not only fragmented, but often also false: "Der Arzt wird leicht geneigt sein, [...] Ansichten und Aussprüche kranker Frauen zu verallgemeinern, wodurch wiederum *ein falsches Bild* entsteht" (4; emphasis added). Brühl claims that physicians convey a false image of female experience because they are limited by a particular point of view.

The scientific analysis provided by Runge is finally obscured by the conviction that women and men constitute two separate species. Brupbacher argues emphatically: "Es ist überhaupt traurig, zu sehen, wie wenig man den Mann zum Vergleich heranzieht, wenn man über die Frau spricht. Von 1000 Dingen, die man dann speciell bei der Frau gefunden zu haben glaubt, werden dann wohl verzweifelt wenige bleiben, die wir nicht auch beim Manne zu finden die Gelegenheit haben" (6). He maintains that men and women share an overwhelming majority of similarities and only a few differences. This fact should actually lead to the conclusion that both sexes are compatible with each other and not to its opposite.

In this context, Laqueur's theory of culturally determined "biology of sexual difference" (19) is worth considering. Laqueur asserts that "[s]ex, in both the one-sex and the two-sex worlds, is situational; it is explicable only within the context of battles over gender and power" (11). According to him, the one-sex model, in which male and female genitals are understood as two variations of the same organ, was replaced by the two-sex model in the course of the eighteenth century. Unlike in the one-sex model, in the two sex-model the male and female genitals are understood as "different in kind"[199] and determine social hierarchy. Although, understandably, not familiar with the theories of sex and gender, Brupbacher seems to grasp the social constructivness of sexual differences.

4.5 The Reproductive Body

All of the writers cited above intervene in Runge's construction of femininity and refute his arguments. Dohm points out that reducing women to the reproductive functions makes them mere instruments of male pleasure and procreation. Dohm further argues that by confining women to reproductive functions only, Runge perceives female life not as an end in itself, but rather as a means to somebody else's life (that of her child) or satisfaction (that of her husband). Dohm emphasizes that Runge and most of the medical literature of the time see this annihilation of the female self as natural: "das Weib ist nur ein Werkzeug zur Hervorbringung des eigentlichen Menschen: – des Mannes" ("Die Ritter" 33). Dohm also quotes Placzek, who opposes female medical education because it would lead to "Vernichtung der Weibernatur, die Vernichtung all jener Charaktereigenschaften, die in ihrer Gegensätzlichkeit zu jenen des Mannes den Hauptgrund für magnetische Attraktionskraft der Geschlechter bilden" ("Die Ritter" 47). She shows that preventing women from entering medical schools has much more to do with male fantasies of the female body and female nature than with the good of women. She concludes that both Runge and Placzek are misled by their sexual instinct ("Die Ritter" 48).

According to Brupbacher, the upbringing of young women makes it impossible for them "etwas anderes zu sein als Geschlechtswerkzeug des Mannes" (10).

199 Laqueur refers to this difference as "[s]exual difference in kind, not degree" (6).

Middle-class women are socialized in a way that does not leave them any option besides entering the institution of marriage. They are unable to pursue an alternative way of living. Scientific knowledge as produced and disseminated by Runge provides a basis and justification for this lack of choices because it presents women as suited exclusively for reproduction. Simultaneously, women internalize the male view of their social role. Hence, it is probable "dass der Kinderinstinkt der Frau nur ein Erziehungsprodukt sei" (Brupbacher 6).

As mentioned above, writers responding to Runge intervene in his construction of femininity as reduced to the sexual sphere. They point out that Runge's woman is not even *das Weib*, but rather only *das Weibchen*. Bülow, paraphrasing Runge's verdict about women, states: "Du sollst Weibchen sein und weiter nichts" ("Das Weib" 600). Meyer demonstrates that Runge "den Weibmenschen vollständig und unbedingt mit dem Tierweibchen gleichsetzt" (712) and Dohm asks: "wenn *sie nur* Weibchen ist, braucht sie doch nur ein Männchen. Wozu denn die Institution der Ehe?" ("Die Ritter" 48). All these statements point out that by defining a woman exclusively in terms of her sexuality, Runge excludes her from human civilization. In his pamphlet, a woman becomes merely a reproductive creature and resembles more an animal than a human being.[200]

Brühl points out that as a result of using different categories of analysis for the sexes, Runge does not seem to perceive women as human beings, but to create a subcategory of humans. Women are seen as being one rung down on the evolutionary ladder and an inferior form of the human species. This limited view, determined by the scientific methods of the time and by the cultural construction of femininity, does not allow Runge to see a woman as a human being equal to man. However, she argues, men and women constitute one and the same category of human beings: "Es giebt nur einen Standpunkt, von dem aus sich ein richtiges Urteil über die Natur des Weibes gewinnen lässt. [...] Dieser eine Standpunkt ist *der neutral menschliche*. Das Wesentliche in der Natur des Weibes ist ebenso wie beim Manne die spezifisch menschliche Natur" (Brühl 4). Brühl draws attention to an overarching category that transcends sexual and gender differences, a category that is non-existent in Runge's pamphlet. Consequently, a woman is denied universal human qualities and becomes a different type of a being than a man. Runge participates in creating what Laqueur calls "the epistemic foundation for prescriptive claims about the social order" (6), and Brühl makes us aware of one such claim: "Runge erkennt den natürlichen Beruf der Frau in der Vollziehung der Fortpflanzungsthätigkeit" (5). As a consequence, "*das Weib* braucht für seinen Beruf weder Geist noch Seele, weder Verstand noch Gemüt. Es hat keine Erziehung, keine Ausbildung nötig, es braucht sogar nicht einmal zu arbeiten. Es braucht nur den Mann" (Brühl 5).

Dohm points out that it is the male popular perception of the female body and its physiological functions, and not these processes themselves, that carry

200 The issue of women being reduced to their sexuality will be developed in Chapter Five.

negative consequences for women. For example, she contends that it is not really the issue of a potential absence from work due to a pregnancy to which physicians object. It is the fact of the pregnancy itself: "Fürst Bismarck zog sich, um eines Nervenleidens willen, alljährlich auf einige Wochen nach Parzin zurück, und niemand hat ihn um dessentwillen für ein zum Staatdienst untaugliches Subjekt gehalten" (Dohm, "Die Ritter" 36). The two cases that she evokes have an identical outcome, a temporary absence from professional work. However, what really matters is the reason for this absence. The absence of an important political figure is justified and its cause, "Nervenleiden," does not have any implications for the perception of his professional competence. At the same time, the absence of a woman due to the processes that are foreign to the male body is defined as having debilitating effects on her professional life. This view is echoed by contemporary feminist critics, such as Rosalyn Diprose, who argued that any divergence from the male norm is theoretically constituted as a deviation and practically manifested through "the treatment of pregnant bodies as disabled" (128).

Many other writers argued as well that physiological processes do not influence a woman's life as negatively as Runge maintains. Bülow, for instance, protests against a common view of womanhood:

> Krankheit, Schmerzen, Siechthum, wohin wir uns auch wenden! Erfüllen wir unseren einzigen Beruf, so setzen wir uns den schweren Gefahren aus und lebenslangem Siechthum. Erfüllen wir ihn nicht, so verkommen wir erst recht. Dennoch sind wir zu nichts Anderem geschaffen und taugen zu nichts Anderem. Ich kann mir weder eine solche Grausamkeit bei Gott noch einen solchen Missgriff bei der Natur vorstellen. Ein solches Jammerwesen ins Leben zu setzen, wäre weder natürlich noch göttlich, sondern satanisch. ("Das Weib" 597)

Similarly, Dohm points out that physicians present woman as "mater dolorosa" by equating female existence with pain and renunciation. As mentioned above, Runge perceives womanhood itself as a sickness that manifests itself through physiological processes and their accompanying side effects. Dohm emphasizes that, according to Runge, a woman is "krank, nichts als eine große Wunde im Weltall" ("Die Ritter" 36) and that, seen from this perspective, "wir armen Kranken wider willen thäten wirklich am besten – wie das verwundete Tier sich ins Dickicht verkriecht – in Kinder-, Schlaf- und Wochenstuben einzig und allein den Kultus unseres Geschlechts zu treiben" ("Die Ritter" 36). While the female physiological functions are imagined by men as incapacitating and uncanny, women experience these natural processes only as "ein paar schmerzensvolle Stunden" (Brühl 11). However, the popular belief in the incapacitating effects of female sexuality made its way into both medical/scientific discourses as well as into the fictional literature and visual arts at the end of the nineteenth century.

Bram Dijkstra documents the portrayal of different visions of femininity in the visual arts of the Fin-de-Siècle in his book *Idols of Perversity. Fantasies of Feminine Evil in Fin-de-Siècle Culture.* Two particular themes in the visual arts, "the cult of feminine invalidism" (*Idols* 25-37) and "the collapsing woman" (*Idols* 64-82), parallel Runge's view of the incapacitating effects of female sexuality. Dijkstra traces a peculiar fascination with the materiality and weakness of the female body in paintings of the late nineteenth century. He points to a significant number of paintings portraying women "as if weighted down by the sheer rotund volume of her material existence, the collapsing woman simply could not seem to manage to keep herself upright. The very effort of living seemed to exhaust her" (Dijkstra, *Idols* 70). According to Dijkstra, this cult is a manifestation of "[t]he esthetic, psychological, and ideological fascination which the theme of the dying or physically spent woman as martyr held for males of the late nineteenth century" (*Idols* 34). In his discussion of Charlotte Perkins Gilman's *The Yellow Wallpaper*, Dijkstra points out that there is an "immediate link [...] between the male creation of [...] the principles of the cult of invalidism, the physicians' encouragement of that cult, and the increasing incidence of madness in women" (*Idols* 36).

The similarity of this statement to Dohm's arguing her need to find an intellectual activity in order to preserve her sanity is striking. Dohm's statement leads one to conclude that physicians such as Runge participate in creating and reinforcing the idea of woman as being inherently ill.[201] The feminine principle becomes almost the uncanny, even for a gynecologist such as Runge. Brühl also hints at the perception of femininity as both destructive and flawed. Ridiculing the notion of inherent female imperfection, she asks rhetorically: "Glaubt der Herr Professor wirklich, der Verstand und die Hände des Mannes arbeiten vollkommener als die Gebärmutter der Frau?" (Brühl 11-12). She exposes such theories as socially and/or (pseudo) scientifically constructed. Therefore they are only relatively and not universally valid. Hence, an exact opposite portrayal is possible:

> Runge hätte, wenn er konsequent wäre, etwa so sprechen müssen: "Die Organisation des Weibes für seinen Beruf ist zweifellos eine *vollkommenere* als die des Mannes für den seinigen. Infolge der unvollkommeneren Organisation des Mannes für seinen Beruf ist ihm ein grösseres Mass von Entsagung und ein grösserer Anspruch an seine Kraft auferlegt als dem Weib. Das Weib geniesst bei Erfüllung seines Berufes anhaltender Mussestunden, es schont seine Hände, seine Sinne und seinen Verstand. Der Mann dagegen muss sein ganzes Selbst einsetzen, seine *ganze Kraft*, seine *Zeit*, oft seine Gesundheit und sein Leben, und was erreicht er trotz alledem im Vergleich zum Weibe? Das Weib bildet im Beruf den Menschen, den Menschen mit seiner ganzen Kraft. [...] Um wie viel mangelhafter

201 See footnote 156.

muss der Mann ausgerüstet sein! Das Weib schafft ohne Mühe göttlich Vollkommenes, der Mann nur Unvollkommenheiten, oft so armes, trauriges Menschenwerk." (Brühl 12).[202]

Brühl does not assert that her claims are true. She only asserts that they are possible conclusions that can be drawn from Runge's premises. By so doing, Brühl illuminates the understanding of human physiology as socially constructed.

One of the main consequences of the theory that women are determined and limited by their sexuality is the alleged lack of cognitive abilities. Dohm and Brühl argue that women are degraded and relegated to an almost "sub-human" category by being denied human characteristics such as these abilities. They become mere reproductive means and as such they need "weder Geist noch Seele, weder Verstand noch Gemüt" (Brühl 5). Brühl opposes the reduction of women to their physiology resulting in the popular notion of women as inferior beings who lack both intellectual and spiritual dimensions. She also shows that by defining women as inherently different from and inferior to men, scientists destroy the basis for demands of women's equality (Brühl 28). Both Brühl and Dohm also insist on a discursive separation of the female body and psyche by denying that gynecologists, such as Runge, possess the necessary expertise to diagnose female intellect and character (Dohm, "Die Ritter" 33; Brühl 4).

Brühl attributes "Streben nach Vollkommenheit" (21) to women and, in so doing, she demonstrates that women are capable of transcending their bodily boundaries. In this drive to perfection, Brühl situates the female self outside the body. She reverses the prevalent perception of women as being equated with their bodies by claiming that the immaterial principle manifests itself in women to a much higher degree than is popularly believed. Brühl refers to this principle as "die hohe seelische Kraft" or "die höhere geistige Kraft" (23). She concludes "dass das geistige Gewicht in der Natur der Frau gegenüber dem körperlichen mindestens ebenso schwer in die Wageschale fällt wie beim Manne" (Brühl 24). Women who work intellectually provide good examples. These women, even if they are not married and do not have children, do not show any signs of becoming "old spinsters." Hence, it is the intellectual, and not the physiological reproductive activity, that gives meaning to women's lives. According to Bülow, women can use their spiritual and physical energy in any way they want without limiting themselves to being wives and mothers: "Diese Kräfte sind vorhanden und können in Arbeit umgesetzt werden, wenn sie für das ursprüngliche Ziel keine Verwendung fanden" ("Das Weib" 598). Bülow further asserts "daß die Erfüllung des Naturberufes allein keineswegs eine glückliche Entfaltung des Weibes sichert" ("Das Weib" 598-99). The treatment she suggests for women's "inherent" illness is different than the one Runge advocates: "Gebt ihren Gedanken Arbeit und ihren

202 This passage is reminiscent of the essay "If Men Could Menstruate" by Gloria Steinem (*Outrageous Acts and Everyday Rebellions*. New York: Henry Holt, 1995. 366-369).

Kräften freie Entfaltung, – und der Hausdrache folgt der alten Jungfer ins Reich der Schatten" (Bülow, "Das Weib" 599).

It is noteworthy that most of Runge's adversaries agree with him on the issue of gender-specific personality and character traits. Unlike Runge, however, they argue that these characteristics are not biologically determined, but rather consequences of women's position in society. Brupbacher, for instance, differentiates between "dem Menschen als physiologischem Menschen, und dem Menschen, wie er durch die Erziehung modifiziert ist" (Brupbacher 4). Nonetheless, the writers responding to Runge do not seem to contradict his assertion that women are prone to certain gender-specific negative traits such as "Gefallsucht" and "Unwahrhaftigkeit" (Brühl 9) as such, but rather they deny that these negative traits are biologically determined. On the contrary, the specific negative traits to which Runge refers are results of particular upbringing, and not a natural inclination. Brupbacher explains the female focus on physical appearance and the desire for male attention as follows: "Es ist also kaum das Streben nach dem anderen Geschlecht beim Weib ein für sich grösseres, sondern Erziehung, Nichtsthun, die Unmöglichkeit, sich selbst zu erhalten und die durch die Prostitution sexuell schon befriedigten Männer sind es, die die Frau veranlassen, den Mann durch alle möglichen Mittel anzuziehen" (11). Brupbacher, Dohm, and Bülow explain the alleged female tendency to lie and cheat in a similar way: "Ungeachtet der hinfälligen Beweisführung bleibt aber die Thatsache bestehen, daß die Frauen listiger und unehrlicher sind als die Männer. Nur ist die Ursache eine ganz andere. [...] Die Frauen sind unwahr geworden, weil sie als die Schwächeren unterdrückt und geknechtet worden sind" (Bülow, "Das Weib" 599-600). Dohm[203] and Brupbacher[204] express similar opinions.

4.6 Modes of Control of the Female Body

In this section I investigate regulatory mechanisms inherent in gender models of the nineteenth century that uphold particular gender relations: bourgeois moral codes, the concept of the inherent male physical brutality, and the notion of female virtue as external and internal means of control. Writers responding to Runge thematize the question of internal and external means by which women are controlled and by which gender models are held in place. Dohm discusses the

---

203 "Ich halte es auch für wahrscheinlich, daß Frauen mehr lügen und trügen, als Männer, einfach aus dem Grunde, weil sie in geistiger und wirtschaftlicher Abhängigkeit leben. Der Unfreie ist immer lügenhafter, als der Freie. Der dauernde Zwiespalt zwischen des Weibes eigenster Natur und der Konvenienz ist ein trefflicher Nährboden für Heuchelei und allerlei Hintertreppenpolitik" ("Die Ritter" 48).

204 "Nehmen wir nun an, sie [die Lügenhaftigkeit] bestehe bei der Frau unzweifelhaft, wie Runge sagt [...]. Es ist eine alte Thatsache und selbstverständlich, dass der Unterdrückte mehr lügt, mehr lügen muss, da ihm von seinem Herrn der gerade Weg verwehrt wird" (Brupbacher 8-9).

prevalent moral standards as a way to control women's behavior. Because these moral standards are deeply ingrained in each individual's consciousness it is very difficult to challenge them. Dohm, however, attempts to contest their very nature.

Dohm reminds her readers of Runge's assertion that the physicality of the female body ("Physis") ("Die Ritter" 33) is the main obstacle to higher education for women, and she also points out that Runge tries to forestall a challenge to his theories when he states that the public discussion of female bodily experience is inappropriate and indecent. Dohm points out that Runge is using the argument of propriety in order to silence women: "Es wäre auch geradezu unehrlich, wenn die Frauen das Hauptargument ihrer Gegner unter dem Vorwand, daß es sich nicht schicke, davon zu reden, *unterschlagen* wollten" ("Die Ritter" 33). Her statement is important because it puts the finger on the normative function of the codes of bourgeois morality and propriety. They are employed to uphold the established gender order. Similarly, Bülow emphasizes that the history of self-expression and self-governance has been very different for men and women: "Während der Mann seit Jahrhunderten in der Lage gewesen ist, sich über sich selbst zu äußern, verschloß die Sitte der Frau den Mund" ("Das Weib" 596). Hence, she exposes the notions of morality and propriety to be regulatory modes of gender relations and repressive guardians of the established female role as wife and mother.

In addition, Dohm points out that references to gallantry or so-called good manners are often used in relation to the "Woman Question" as an excuse not to acknowledge the opposing arguments and to silence women. She refers to Runge's statement, "Wir Männer [...] haben uns gewöhnt, das Weib zu beurteilen durch die Maske der Galanterie" ("Die Ritter" 34), in order to show that such an understanding of gender relations negates the possibility of honesty and equality. She also demonstrates that there is another aspect of male chivalry. According to her, men demonstrate their politeness mainly towards attractive women: "Männer pflegen sich doch nur jungen und hübschen Damen gegenüber galant zu erweisen. Häßlichen, ältlichen oder alten gegenüber befleißigen sich gerade die Ärzte viel eher der Unhöflichkeit und Grobheit, wenn nicht durch äußere Umstände gebotene Rücksichtnahmen ihrer Unhöflichkeit Zügel anlegen" (Dohm, "Die Ritter" 34). Gynecologists are much more inclined to talk "[v]on ihren [der Frauen] physischen Reizen und Nichtreizen" than "von ihren psychischen" (Dohm, "Die Ritter" 34). She indicates that in the first place the gynecologist's function is to examine the woman's body and not her brain. Additionally she hints at the male tendency to dismiss the intellectual dimension in women in general.

According to Dohm, chivalry turns out to be only a mask, put on with a particular goal in mind since "der Mann neben und hinter der Galanterie auch brutal gegen das Weib sei" ("Die Ritter" 34). She responds directly to Runge's assertion that male physical brutality is a biologically determined feature and points out that women suffer the consequences of this theory: "Naive Schlußfolgerung, die Runge aus der Brutalität des Mannes zieht! Weil der Mann brutal ist, sperre man das Weib ein, damit er ihr nichts thun kann! [...] Ja, wir brauchten also gar keinen

Schutz, wenn der Mann nicht brutal wäre! Ließe sich denn nicht die Brutalität des Mannes abschaffen?" (Dohm, "Die Ritter" 34). The external mode of control there is male physical force.

Because Runge sees male brutality as biologically determined, he reinforces the notion of its inevitability. In response to this claim, Bülow asserts that men enjoy unlimited freedom at the cost of women's liberty and her confinement to the private sphere. She further paraphrases Runge in order to reveal what, according to her, is his hidden agenda: "Weil das Weib schwach [...] und weil der Mann brutal ist, müssen wir im Interesse des Weibes die Frauenemanzipation mit voller Energie bekämpfen. Das bedeutet nicht viel mehr als ein bewusstes, gewolltes Aufrechterhalten der Schwäche des Weibes und der Brutalität des Mannes" (Bülow, "Das Weib" 601). Bülow reveals Runge's underlying unwillingness to consider potential changes in gender roles in order to improve the lives of women because they would result in new limitations imposed on the male's existence. Hence, what Runge defines as a natural gender order, Bülow exposes as the socially constructed inequality of the sexes, which she describes as "die Errichtung von unnatürlichen Mauern und Schranken" (Bülow, "Das Weib" 601). For her, the traditional split into male and female realms is by no means naturally determined; it is "eine *keineswegs naturgemäße* Einwickelung und Abschließung der 'Dame' gerade in den oberen Schichten" (Bülow, "Das Weib" 598; emphasis added). In order to demonstrate that the core of the resentment towards any conscious changes of the established gender models is the male's advantageous position and not the woman's good, Dohm raises the issue of the female corset that has tangible negative effects on women's health: "Warum agitieren die Ärzte nicht insgesamt gegen das Korsett, und was sonst in der Frauentracht gesundheitsstörend ist?" ("Die Ritter" 46).

According to Bülow and Brühl, the oppressive gender system was developed throughout the ages based on male physical strength. Brühl emphasizes that the privileged male position in society is nothing but "das Recht des Stärkeren in seiner untersten Deutung" (28). Explaining the consequences of the oppressive gender system for women Bülow argues:

> Darum, weil der Mann mit dem Recht des Stärkeren dekretierte: "Ihr Frauen sollt nur Weibchen sein, das Andere wollen wir allein besorgen", darum ist es geschehen, daß sich Menschenweib zu merkwürdiger Einseitigkeit entwickeln mußte. Statt sein Menschenthum zu entfalten und zu gestalten mußte es immer mehr sein Sinnen auf das Locken und Umgarnen des herrschenden Männchens richten und wurde so wirklich immer mehr zum Nur-Weibchen. ("Das Weib" 600)

The dogmatic view of gender differences and of specific male and female roles derived from this stance restricts the unlimited potential and distorts the real character and natural abilities of women. According to Bülow, women have internalized and appropriated this very limited and distorted view of gender models. Many women, for example, suffer if they cannot fulfill what was defined for them as a typically feminine existence. But they suffer not because a different type of existence is against their nature, but because they were socialized in a certain way: "Der [...] bekannte und viel verlachte Typus [die alte Jungfrau] entstand aber nicht dadurch, daß das Weib seinen Naturberuf nicht erfüllen konnte, sondern dadurch, daß es diese Natur-Aufgabe als einzigen wahren Beruf des Weibes aufzufassen gelehrt worden war" (Bülow, "Das Weib" 598). Bülow, however, indicates that she and her contemporaries are witnessing an important shift in gender relations: "Die überzählige, unverwerthete Frau wird sich ihrer Kräfte bewußt und verlangt, sie uneingeschränkt ausleben zu dürfen" ("Das Weib" 598). Here she addresses the concept of the New Woman thematized in the nineteenth-century feminist press and other publications.[205] Her statement indicates that there is a profound sense of an ongoing transformation of social consciousness that produces new understandings of gender models.

205 The concept of the New Woman will be discussed in Chapter Five.

5 Against Pornographic Imagination: The Autonomous Female Body

[T]he boundary between 'pornography' and other imagery framed within a masculine gaze is not easy, if at all possible, to define.

Jane M. Ussher[206]

[T]he secret message in the pornographic revelation of beauty [...] is to rob the female body of both its natural power and its spiritual presence. [...] The mystery of the female body is revealed to be nothing more than flesh, and flesh under culture's control.

Susan Griffin[207]

5.1 Introduction: Reactions to Paul Julius Möbius

In 1900, Paul Julius Möbius, a Leipzig neuropsychiatrist, published a short pamphlet of twenty-six pages with the scandalous and provocative title, *Über den physiologischen Schwachsinn des Weibes.*[208] The text became a bestseller, was republished several times, and made its author famous. By the time of Möbius' death in 1907, the eighth edition had been published and consisted of approximately two hundred pages.[209] Each new edition included a revised introduction and an appendix comprised of responses to the text that had been received since its previous publication.[210] Divided into four categories, it included the critical responses themselves: positive and negative reviews, excerpts from letters by physicians and scientists, and finally the female responses.[211] The book continued to be published posthumously, reaching its twelfth edition in 1922. In addition, the pamphlet has been reissued in 1977, 1990, 2000, and 2001 at the Matthes & Seitz publishing house. As already indicated, the reception of the pamphlet at the time of its initial publication was twofold. A large number of reviewers focused on the lack of scientific validity of the text and on its demeaning character. Many others, however, perceived it as a scientifically based and convincing piece of writing. Whether the text is scientific or not, it mirrors gender politics and the struggles of the time and, in Mary Caputi's words, it "encapsulates the nexus of power

206 Ussher 245.

207 Griffin 33; also qtd. in Ussher 178.

208 See also Thorson's discussion of Möbius' text 13-17.

209 See also Schiller 98.

210 See also Schiller 98 and Thorson 13.

211 The first edition (1900) consisted of 26 pages, the second edition (1901) of 34 pages, the third edition (1901) of 93 pages, the fourth edition (1902) of 101 pages, the fifth edition (1903) of 123 pages, the sixth edition (1904) of 131 pages, the seventh edition (1905) of 140 pages, and the eighth edition (1905) of 212 pages.

relations surrounding gender and sexuality as conceived within our culture" (1).[212] The title of the book, the fact that it was written by a respected scientist, as well as the publication and reception history raise many questions pertaining to gender politics and the role of science and popular culture in reinforcing a particular gender ideology. Before I discuss these questions, however, I would like to give a brief overview of reactions to the text that situate *Über den physiologischen Schwachsinn des Weibes* both outside of and within a scientific discourse.

Among the first group to respond to the text were many intellectuals and activists campaigning for women's education. Dohm, for example, responded to the third edition of the book in 1901 as follows: "Nachdem ich die Schrift gelesen, wunderte ich mich, daß sie nicht schon die zehnte Auflage erlebt hat, amüsant wie sie ist" ("Randglossen" 18). According to Dohm, the book belongs to "den lächerlichen Mißgriffen" ("Randglossen" 18) that will eventually contribute to the victory of the women's movement because it contains self-evident nonsense. In her article, "Ein Retter vom Geist," Martha Asmus emphasizes "Mangel an Ernst seiner [Möbius'] Untersuchung" (235). One of Asmus' main arguments is precisely that one cannot take Möbius seriously. She quotes specific passages to support her claim. One example she quotes from *Über den physiologischen Schwachsinn des Weibes* reads as follows: "In den Zeiten politischer Unsicherheit hat man mit Schrecken die Ungerechtigkeit und Grausamkeit der Weiber kennen gelernt, ebenso an den Weibern, die unglücklicherweise zur Herrschaft gekommen sind ..." (Asmus 237). For Asmus, this passage is ridiculous. She comments: "Freilich muß er [Möbius] selbst in der alten Weltgeschichte unbewandert sein und z.B. die römischen Cäsaren nicht kennen" (Asmus 237). Obviously the tendency to cruelty and injustice cannot be reasonably attributed to women to a higher degree than it can be ascribed to men. Similarly, Frieda von Bülow points out that the only reasonable reaction to Möbius' book is "nur lächelnd den Kopf schütteln" ("Schwachsinn des Weibes" 17). Ladislaus Gumplowicz indicates that even his own response to Möbius' text seems silly due to the nature of the pamphlet itself and its lack of serious scientific basis: "Es ist nicht meine Schuld, wenn die Sache humoristisch wird. Herr Dr. Möbius hat es sich stellenweise doch wohl etwas zu leicht gemacht" (910). Clearly, remarks such as "Häßlich heißt ja hassenswert" (Möbius, *Schwachsinn* 51) could not have been taken seriously in terms of scientific or even pseudoscientific validity even at the turn of the twentieth century. However, statements like the one quoted exemplify the specific gender ideology behind Möbius' text that I will discuss in this chapter.

As mentioned above, not all reviews were negative. Many readers actually embraced Möbius' view of female nature precisely because of its ideological underpinnings. Others overlooked the evident misogyny and/or classified the text as scientific. Richarda Huch, for instance, fails to notice the highly demeaning tone of the pamphlet:

---

212 In the quoted passage, Caputi defines pornography in our culture. However, it can be also applied to characterize accurately Möbius' text.

> In neuerer Zeit haben die Schriften des bekannten Psychiaters Möbius über die Frau, in denen er das moderne Streben, die Intelligenz der Frau auszubilden, für verderblich erklärt, ein gewisses Aufsehen erregt und zum Teil Entrüstung hervorgerufen, letzteres, wie mir scheint, nicht ganz mit recht, da die Absicht des Verfassers gut und auch seine Meinung über die Frauen, sofern man sich nur an die Sache hält, nicht kränkend ist. (746)

Among the positive responses that Möbius included in the later editions of the book, there are many that do not deny the scientific validity of the text:

> Ursprünglich *war der Aufsatz nur für medizinische Kreise bestimmt und in der "Sammlung zwangsloser Abhandlungen aus dem Gebiete der Nerven- und Geisteskrankheiten" erschienen.* Erst die dritte Auflage bildet nun eine selbständige Broschüre, wohl weil der Verfasser in einem sehr langen Vorworte eine Reihe von Mißverständnissen aufzuklären und durch neue Beiträge das Verständnis für das, was er eigentlich will, zu erleichtern versucht. (Möbius, *Schwachsinn* 128; emphasis added)[213]

The author of this review implies that the pamphlet was misunderstood by those who did not have medical training. Consequently, Möbius was forced to provide additional explanations in order to defend his work. Although the author of the review mentions logical and procedural errors in the pamphlet, he emphasizes that "die Abhandlung den Anspruch einer rein wissenschaftlichen macht" (Möbius, *Schwachsinn* 128). Wulff Oldenburg's review cited by Möbius reads: "In dieser sehr interessanten Arbeit *weist der bekannte Verfasser in höchst genialer Weise nach,* daß das Weib [...] karger mit Geistesgaben versehen ist, als der Mann" (Möbius, *Schwachsinn* 131; emphasis added). These are only a few examples of the many enthusiastic reviews that treat Möbius' text seriously and do not deny the scientific validity of his undertaking.

When the collected works of Möbius appeared after his death, the text on female physiological feeble-mindedness was not included. Ernst Jentsch, the editor, wrote an introduction and a biography of Möbius for this collected edition and commented on this specific text as follows:

> [Den] Ausdruck [...] des morphologischen Unterschiedes zwischen Mann und Weib [...] [nannte] Möbius den "physiologischen Schwachsinn" des Weibes [...]. Die wesentliche Bedeutung dieses Sachverhalts für gewisse Tagesfragen veranlaßte ihn zu der

213 An article published originally in *Wissenschaftliche Beilage zur Germania,* 8 Aug. 1901. Möbius does not provide the title of the article.

Abfassung der Abhandlung, die diesen Titel führt und seitdem weithin bekannt geworden ist [...]. Da man in größeren Kreisen von Möbius' Arbeitsgebiet und Arbeitsweise nichts wußte, so faßte man diese allenthalben zunächst affektiv auf und hielt sie für eine Tendenzschrift, man glaubte dadurch bestimmte moderne Ideale gefährdet und hörte sozusagen nur das Nein dabei heraus." (*Beiträge zur Lehre* 27)

Although Jentsch tries to impose some kind of scientific validity onto the text, he does not explain why it was not included in the collected works. The only reasonable explanation seems to be precisely the lack of scientific value. On the other hand, however, the seemingly earnest tone of the pamphlet; references to scientists such as Bischoff, Rüdiger, and Lombroso;[214] and the attempt to deliver a theory of femininity seem to attest to the seriousness of the undertaking.

The text itself leaves the reader puzzled as to the intentions of the author. On many occasions, one is actually inclined to think that Möbius delivered a parody of all previous texts on femininity and intended this pamphlet only as an entertaining piece, even if in bad taste. Regardless of whether this text emerged as a serious attempt to define femininity or whether it was only an effort to make the author famous, it exemplifies a particular view of femininity that was taken seriously enough at the time of its publication to generate a significant number of responses.

The second part of the pamphlet, in which Möbius reviews and discusses responses to his book, gives the reader the impression that the author is rather amused and pleased by all the uproar. Francis Schiller, the author of a monograph on Möbius, explains the shocking title of the book. When approached by a friend and questioned about the title, Möbius replied: "Oh well, that was only to boost the sales!" (Strümpell qtd. in Schiller 98). Schiller further points out:

> Nobody will be, or was, surprised that in the suffragette age, Möbius' book became a *success de scandale,* or that it made the author known in circles rather removed from neurology, psychiatry, biography, and philosophy. As the feminist movement was reaching its first apex, such a book could only be a regular success with the conservative lay and medical press. (103)

Schiller's observation seems to confirm that Möbius' primary intent was to generate publicity and additional income and not to deliver a scientific text. Schiller also points out that the book was a product of its time, because Möbius did "voice the average opinion about [women]" (101) and because the perception of female

---

214 Möbius references three case studies that claimed to prove female intellectual inferiority, the book *Das Weib als Verbrecherin und Prostituierte* by Ferrero and Lombroso, as well as research by Bischoff and Rüdinger.

intellectual inferiority was "a cultural observation of the period" (99). However, the book would not have generated so many responses had Möbius voiced only average sentiments on women. Both Schiller and Jentsch fail to acknowledge that Möbius' text went much further than merely asserting "that the average female mind did not measure up to the male's" (Schiller 99).

In 1902 the feminist magazine *Die Frau* published an article by Ika Freudenberg entitled "Oda Olberg contra Dr. Moebius." The article was a review of Oda Olberg's book *Das Weib und der Intellectualismus* in which Olberg not only addressed Möbius' pamphlet, but also delivered a sophisticated theory of culture. In her article, Freudenberg juxtaposed both texts and both authors as follows:

> Wenn ein namhafter Gelehrter eine wissenschaftliche Abhandlung schreibt, so wird man erwarten, den Gegenstand darin mit großer Gründlichkeit und von allen Seiten betrachtet zu finden, unter gewissenhafter Abgrenzung der Begriffssphären, unter genauer Berücksichtigung aller in Frage kommenden Nebengebiete und aller möglichen Einwände; dabei mit stolzer Vermeidung aller Banalitäten, die an den Unterhaltungston von Klub oder Biertisch erinnern könnten – kurz im ganzen mit einer strengen Ernsthaftigkeit und so ganz und gar nicht populär, daß die große Masse, die zum Vergnügen liest, einer solchen Lektüre in weitem Bogen aus dem Wege geht. Und wenn eine Frau ohne akademische Bildung über eine wissenschaftliche Frage schreibt, zumal über eine, die sie selbst aufs tiefste berührt, so wird man auf Schritt und Tritt merken, daß es ihr an jener Objektivität mangelt [...]. Eine solche Frauenschrift wird durch und durch tendenziös sein, d.h. sie wird die Dinge unwillkürlich so zurechtlegen, daß eine bestimmte Ansicht herausspringen muß. Sie wird es verstehen für eine wissenschaftliche Arbeit einen Titel zu finden, der geeignet ist, Interesse und Neugier zu erwecken. Und das Endergebnis wird sein, daß ein solches Werkchen hernach in allen Schaufenstern hängt und daß der darauf geklebte bunte Zettel, der *abermals eine neue Auflage* ankündigt, in Gemeinschaft mit dem verheißungsvollen Titel eine geradezu fascinierende Wirkung ausübt. [...] Die Broschüre [...] von Oda Olberg als Entgegnung auf Dr. Moebius [...] beweist, daß es sich auch einmal gerade umgekehrt verhalten kann! (620)

Freudenberg alludes to a certain shift regarding functions, expectations, and positions in the scientific and popular discourses. This passage illustrates two important developments in the context of the debate about the admission of women to higher education. On the one hand, it reflects a change in the mode of the debate from scientific to personal or philosophical that is exemplified by Möbius' text.

On the other hand, this passage also implies that women's intellectual development can indeed measure up to male intellectual abilities or that it can even supersede them. In her text, Olberg not only speaks from a position of authority based on her gender and specific physiological functions particular to the female body, but she also manifests significant scientific expertise. Freudenberg's argument also confirms that the primary function of Möbius' text was not a scientific one, but rather that the pamphlet was intended primarily as a demeaning piece of writing.

I argue that *Über den physiologischen Schwachsinn des Weibes* is not a book about female feeble-mindedness, as the title suggests, but rather about male (heterosexual) pleasure, objectification of women, and gender power relations.[215] The fact that the book was written and published during the early phases of women's struggle for equality magnifies this meaning. In addition, I propose that Möbius' text fulfilled a twofold function. On the one hand, it served as a cultural manifesto that advocated reversing the emancipatory trends of modernity. As such, it reaffirmed the patriarchal world order with its traditionally established values, gender norms, and boundaries. On the other hand, it reiterated male subjectivity by creating an image of women that was based entirely on their objectification and humiliation in the context of their embodied sexuality. In this regard, I would label Möbius' text as pornographic. Although it does not convey explicitly sexual images, it contains the elements typical of a pornographic depiction of women: emphasis on particular body parts; reduction of female humanity and individuality to the material body; a demeaning attitude toward or derogatory portrayal of women; and imagined female inferiority, be it physical, intellectual, or moral.[216] I contend that precisely these two functions of the text provoked both the positive and the negative responses and contributed to its popularity. In addition, *Über den physiologischen Schwachsinn des Weibes* is a culmination of the misogynistic (pseudo) scientific texts that grew out of the debate about women's medical education.

5.2 Möbius' Text as a Cultural Manifesto

Möbius' text and the responses it generated constitute the last phase of the debate about women's admission to medical schools. Although Möbius does not discuss the issue of medical education for women in depth, he indirectly acknowledges this debate to be the catalyst for his text. Möbius was aware that at the beginning of the twentieth century many women had already been admitted to universities in

215 In her book *Voluptuous Yearnings*, Mary Caputi summarizes the main arguments made by feminists against pornography. She hints at these three elements (male [heterosexual] pleasure, objectification of women, and power) as the main elements of many definitions of pornography (1-2; 12; 15-16).

216 See Subchapter 5.3. The notion of pornography discussed in this chapter refers to pornography aimed at heterosexual men.

Germany and many successfully studied and practiced medicine. Therefore, he changed the focus of the discussion and claimed that the admission of women to medical schools was not the real issue:

> Die Ärzte haben sich vielfach über die Forderung der Weiber, zur Medizin zugelassen zu werden, erregt. Vielleicht ist die Sache nicht so wichtig. Einerseits ist nicht zu leugnen, daß die weiblichen Geistesfähigkeiten zur Erlernung der Medizin ausreichen, und daß gelegentlich weibliche Ärzte, wenn sie gehörig geleitet und beaufsichtigt werden, nützlich sein können (z. B. in mohamedanischer Bevölkerung), andererseits werden sich doch nur recht wenige Mädchen dem Studium zuwenden, immer weniger, je mehr die Sache an "Aktualität" verliert, und diese wenigen werden solche sein, die für ihren weiblichen Beruf sowieso nicht recht tauglich sind. Also wenn auch die Medizin wie die Weiber selbst vom weiblichen Studium nicht viel Nutzen haben werden, es kommt nicht sehr viel darauf an. (*Schwachsinn* 42)

Faced with the overwhelming evidence that women are indeed capable of studying medicine, Möbius dismisses the struggle for admission to universities as a fashionable trend that will end as soon as it loses its novel allure. Therefore, Möbius appeals to physicians to disregard women's attempts to study and practice medicine and to focus instead on the lack of female cognitive abilities and its consequences:

> Viel wichtiger scheint mir das zu sein, *daß die Ärzte sich eine klare Vorstellung von dem weiblichen Gehirn- oder Geisteszustande verschaffen, daß sie die Bedeutung und den Wert des weiblichen Schwachsinnes begreifen,* und daß sie alles tun, was in ihren Kräften steht, um im Interesse des menschlichen Geschlechts die widernatürlichen Bestrebungen der "Feministinnen" zu bekämpfen. Es handelt sich hier um die Gesundheit des Volkes, die durch die Verkehrtheit der "modernen Frauen" gefährdet wird. (*Schwachsinn* 42)

With its nationalistic rhetoric,[217] the quoted passage is a call for action to combat the "unnatural" efforts of women's emancipation. Möbius advocates a specific view of female cognitive abilities that justifies his position and makes it seemingly the only reasonable standpoint. In addition, the passage sets the tone for the entire pamphlet which is a plea for the reversal of modern emancipatory developments.[218]

---

217 Thorson uses the same phrase, "nationalistic rhetoric," in relation to Möbius (15).

218 Schmersahl maintains that many scientists made a connection between modernity and women transgressing gender norms. She writes: "Besonders aus einer kulturpessimistischen

The text is a public declaration of the author's desire to put an end to what he saw as feminism and it has a programmatic character. It demands concrete action and justifies this call on the basis of a misogynistic ideology. Hence, it becomes a cultural manifesto reflecting one of the main trends of the time. Möbius insists that "female feeble-mindedness" is both inevitable and necessary for a well-functioning society. He states: "[D]er weibliche Schwachsinn [ist] nicht nur vorhanden, sondern auch *notwendig*, er ist nicht nur ein physiologisches Faktum, sondern auch ein physiologisches *Postulat*" (*Schwachsinn* 41; emphasis added). His is a call to sustain socially or even to create female feeble-mindedness by keeping women at home away from the public sphere of influence and by denying them access to higher education. Many writers responding to Möbius grasped the programmatic character of his text. Olberg, for example, reads the text as advancing "geistige Inferiorität als Postulat" (86-100). Dohm points out that Möbius' main goal is to uphold the subjugation of women and not to establish any type of scientific truth: "Wie? Die Frauen bemühen sich, ihren niedrigen Charakter zu veredeln, sich ihrer Tierähnlichkeit allmählich zu entäußern, und die Möbiusse, anstatt ihnen die helfende Hand zu reichen, stoßen sie in die Tiefe der Tierheit zurück? Wer den Menschen hindert, sich aufwärts zu entwickeln, ist kulturfeindlich" ("Randglossen" 36). Möbius attempts to uphold the privileged male position in society and fights against any attempts at gender equality. In her response, Olberg explains what she understands to be the underlying ideology of Möbius' manifesto, that is, that the pursuit of happiness should be reserved only for men. Women's happiness is defined by social standards; it consists of keeping house and of having children. Any attempt at finding satisfaction in a different sphere is considered to be a sign of degeneration because it aims at transgressing strictly defined gender roles.[219] Olberg emphasizes that although every human being wants to be happy, women are not allowed to pursue this goal. According to her, it is "eine widrige mittelalterliche Auffassung [...], die in Freude, Wohlsein und Lust etwas Böses sieht, die aus der impotenten Gier der Krankhaftigkeit heraus die Freudigkeit, die Gesundheit ist und Gesundheit bringt, als Sünde verdammt" (Olberg 87). Olberg further claims that Möbius demands a new type of renunciation, namely "die intellectuelle Enthaltsamkeit des Weibes" (90). This new philosophy replaced the older "Ueberschätzung der sexuellen Unberührtheit" (Olberg 90).

---

und zivilisationskritischen Sicht deuteten viele Autoren das 'Mannweib' als sichtbares Zeichen für die Krankhaftigkeit der Moderne" (325). She further explains that Möbius was one of these physicians who had a quite pessimistic view of modern civilization: "So setzte Möbius Zivilisation mit Nervosität, der Auflösung der Geschlechtercharaktere und damit dem Auftreten von Mannweibern gleich" (325). Weiershausen, too, poins to the connection between modernity and women transgressing gender norms by arguing that, in several fictional works of the time, the female student was associated with modernity (214).

219 See footnote 23.

Möbius ends his text with a plea for a much milder penal code for women because they are naturally inclined to engage in criminal behavior: "Je mehr das Weib aus dem Schutze des Hauses heraustritt, um so leichter wird sie mit den Gesetzen in Konflikt kommen" (*Schwachsinn* 45). Hence, he suggests a different penal code for women who should be treated more leniently than men due to their feeble-mindedness (*Schwachsinn* 44-45). This is, of course, not an appeal for a better social position for women, but yet another declaration of women's inability to make the right choices and of the necessity to strictly control women's behavior. Hence, this statement attempts to reaffirm the long-established gender roles and limits of socially acceptable behavior as well as women's dependency on men. With this claim, Möbius reiterates the traditional understanding of women as irrational creatures.

Ladislaus Gumplowicz adopted the programmatic tone of Möbius' pamphlet and responded with an opposing manifesto that reaffirmed the need for a change in traditional gender roles and demanded equal rights for women. At the same time, he directly addressed Möbius' claims regarding gender differences. He did not deny that there were profound differences between men and women but argued that these differences do not support inequality. Even differently constituted individuals should have the same rights, privileges, and opportunities available to them:

> Wir fordern gleiches *Recht* für beide Geschlechter. Diese unsere Forderung ist aber keineswegs gleichbedeutend mit der Leugnung der vorhandenen physischen und psychischen Geschlechtsunterschiede. [...] Die Forderung gleichen Rechtes für alle schliesst [...] qualitative Verschiedenheiten des Studiums und Berufes nicht aus, [...] im Gegenteil, jene Forderung kann nur erfüllt werden, indem das Gemeinwesen die qualitativ verschiedenen Bedürfnisse seiner einzelnen Mitglieder durch *entsprechend verschiedene Darbietungen* gleich gut befriedigt. (Gumplowicz 902-903)

He argues that the anatomical and psychological differences between men and women should be considered when establishing equal laws and opportunities. These differences do not exclude equal rights and do not predispose women to a subordinated position. Gumplowicz voices the following demands: "[W]as wir verlangen, ist, dass der Frau ganz ebenso wie dem Manne der Weg offen stehe zu jeglicher Berufstätigkeit, zu der sie die individuelle Befähigung besitzt; dass kein vorhandenes Talent irgend eines Mädchens bloss deshalb zum Verkümmern verurteilt werde, weil dieses Talent in einem Mädchenkopfe steckt" (903). This passage is a plea for a new gender order that would enable Virginia Woolf's well-known "Shakespeare's sister" and Hedwig Dohm's lesser-known "Friederike Schiller" to have the same opportunities as their male counterparts. At a time when profound changes in the understanding of a woman's role in society took place and when the women's movement achieved numerous victories, Möbius' text can be understood as a reactionary attempt to annihilate these developments and to reaffirm traditional limits and boundaries. It is a text with a strong programmatic character in which the author calls for combined efforts of all physicians, if not all men, to uphold the underprivileged female role in society. Since the admission of women to higher education throughout Europe contributed to a new outlook on femininity and helped create more fluid gender boundaries, Möbius' text was perceived by feminists as a violation of and a threat to the new unwritten values.

5.3 Pornographic Imagination

Contemporary discussions of pornography allow me to situate Möbius' text in the framework of what I call the pornographic imagination. Reception of the text at the time of its initial publication in Germany demonstrates that intellectuals such as Johanna Elberskirchen, Hedwig Dohm, Martha Asmus, and Frieda von Bülow made a similar connection and were able to grasp the pornographic ideology underlying the text, although they did not have the extensive theoretical vocabulary of contemporary gender studies to express it. Before I discuss Möbius's text as an example of pornographic imagination, I will give an overview of contemporary feminist views on pornography and define the notion of pornographic imagination.

Susanne Kappeler has demonstrated that one unambiguous definition of pornography does not exist. She argues that "[i]nstead, different discussions identify different characteristic elements as their basis for a discussion of the phenomenon" (1). Kappeler also points out that different groups are concerned with pornography for different reasons, and that in the majority of cases the question of pornography "is being reframed as one of obscenity and censorship or of freedom of expression" (18) and that "[w]omen are defined out of the question" (18). A glance at a standard definition proves her assertion to be correct. The *Oxford English Dictionary*, for example, defines pornography as: "Description of the life, manners, etc., of prostitutes and their patrons; hence, the expression or suggestion of obscene or unchaste subjects in literature or art; pornographic literature or art."[220] Although the etymology of the compound "pornography" leads to the Greek word "pórnē," meaning "prostitute" ("Pornography." *The Barnhart Dictionary of Etymology*), what is missing in this definition is a reference to the role assigned to all women in traditional pornographic texts and images aimed at heterosexual men. Catharine A. MacKinnon and Andrea Dworkin were the first to redefine pornography by focusing on the question of representation of all women, not only prostitutes. The crucial part of their definition reads: "the graphic sexually explicit subordination of women through pictures or words" (MacKinnon 176). This definition coins a new understanding of pornography by changing two

220 Definition also qtd. in Kappeler 155-56.

crucial terms. The words "prostitutes" and "obscene" are dropped and the words "women" and "subordination" are added instead. Hence, a moral question relating to the world of commercialized sexual exchange transforms into an issue of power pertaining to all women. At the same time, a subjective moral judgment ("obscene" and "unchaste") concerned with the content ("description of the life, manners, etc." and "subjects") becomes less relevant. Instead, the question of power relations between the sexes comes into play. MacKinnon spells out this difference by dissociating obscenity from pornography:

> Obscenity [...] is a moral idea, an idea about judgments of good and bad. Pornography, by contrast, is a political practice, a practice of power and powerlessness. Obscenity is ideational and abstract; pornography is concrete and substantive. [...] Obscenity as such probably does little harm. Pornography is integral to attitudes and behaviors of violence and discrimination that define the [...] treatment and status of half the population. (175)

It is important for my discussion of Möbius' text that, from the point of view represented by MacKinnon, Dworkin, Kappeler, and many others, "[p]ornography is not a special case of sexuality; it is a form of representation" (Kappeler 2). It is evident from the quoted passages that, to repeat Kappeler's formulation, "feminist critique is concerned with sexism, not with indecency or obscenity" (25). Feminists "object to the degradation of women in pornography, [not] to the presence of a particular kind of 'sex' in pornographic representations" (Kappeler 102). In her book *Pornography. Men Possessing Women*, Dworkin argues that the primary function of pornography is to assert male subjectivity and to "celebrate male power" (25). In her view, pornography is not about sexual practice itself. Rather, it is about using the female body and sexual practices to reaffirm men's subject position. In order to achieve this aim, woman is turned into an object and degraded. Dworkin claims that "the degradation of women [in pornography] exists in order to postulate, exercise, and celebrate male power. Male power, in degrading women, is first concerned with itself, its perpetuation, expansion, intensification, and elevation" (25). She further argues that "[m]ale supremacy depends on the ability of men to view women as sexual objects" (Dworkin 113). Pornography perpetuates such an ideology of gender relations not only by the sheer depiction of the female body, but rather by suggesting "that the use of the female body for sexual or reproductive purposes is a natural right of men; that the sexual will of men properly and naturally defines the parameters of a woman's sexual being, which is her whole identity" (Dworkin 203). Hence, the key feature of pornography is that it turns women into objects and that it dehumanizes them as a result. At the same time it has a constitutive character. It "constructs the social reality of gender" (MacKinnon 166). MacKinnon suggests that the male sexualized gaze constructs the meaning of women's existence. Men look at women through the prism of their own sexual gratification. This way of seeing connected to the male privileged position gives men the power to assign a specific social role to women, the role of a sexual object. She argues: "[m]en treat women as who they see women as being. Pornography constructs who that is. Men's power over women means that the way men see women defines who women can be. Pornography is that way" (MacKinnon 148).[221] Similarly, pornography "institutionalizes the sexuality of male supremacy" and "constitutes the meaning of that sexuality" (MacKinnon 148).[222]

Many feminist thinkers have pointed out that the ideology underlying pornographic representation of women is not limited to pornography. As a matter of fact, it permeates Western "high" and popular culture as a belief that women's obligation and main purpose of existence is to serve men sexually. This notion, to which some critics refer as "metaphysics of pornography" (Griffin 14) is rooted in the conviction of an inherent male superiority. In her book *Fantasies of Femininity: Reframing the Boundaries of Sex*, Jane M. Ussher elaborates on the connection between pornography and other types of texts and images as follows:

> Despite the absence of subtlety, pornography cannot be separated from every other representation of "woman" frozen in the masculine gaze [...]. For the image of "woman" purveyed in pornography is not unique, it is the extreme end of a continuum. It is perhaps the last bastion of the unfettered masculine gaze, where the influence of "woman" as spectator is absent from the scene and the power of "man" as phallic hero is unthreatened or untamed. In pornography, the process of fetishization and objectification of "woman" we have seen in art and film is merely more obviously played out. It is perhaps the last politically incorrect playground for those who believe in (or fantasize about) the *natural* power of "man" over "woman." (180)

Ussher further detects a specific gender ideology underlying pornography and many other texts and images that is "crudely heterosexist, phallocentric and sympathetic to the fantasies of 'man'" (180). In other words, according to Ussher, men's artistic and non-artistic representations of women are always tainted by their own sexuality. Pornography is different from other representations of women only in degree, not in kind. Kappeler refers to this phenomenon as "the pornographic structure of representation" which she defines as "the systematic objectification of women in the interest of the exclusive subjectification of men" (103). Hence, "the pornographic structure of representation" is not limited to texts and images that contain sexually explicit material as pornography is.

221 Also qtd. in Caputi 16-17.
222 Also qtd. in Caputi 16.

The term I use in relation to Möbius' text, the pornographic imagination, builds on Kappeler's "pornographic structure of representation." I also draw on a term coined by Susan Griffin, "pornographic mind." In addition, my point of reference is the title of an article by Susan Sontag, "The Pornographic Imagination."[223] Before I discuss the notion of the pornographic imagination, I would like to examine briefly the texts by Sontag and Griffin. Sontag defines "the pornographic imagination" as a "form of consciousness" (67) that produces texts "whose primary, exclusive, and overriding preoccupation is with the depiction of sexual 'intentions' and 'activities'" (66) aiming at "inducing sexual excitement" (39). In light of my earlier discussion of feminist analyses of pornography, I approach the notion of the pornographic imagination from a different perspective. Specifically, I focus on the representation of women in relation to men, a representation which is determined by the male subject position and by the male (hetero) sexual fantasy. However, Sontag mentions three important characteristics of a pornographic representation that I find useful for my reading of Möbius' text. She points out that the characters in a pornographic scenario are always interchangeable (Sontag 53) and "endowed with neither will nor intelligence" (Sontag 53). In addition, there is a permanent gap "between one's existence as a full human being and one's existence as a sexual being" (Sontag 58).

In her book *Pornography and Silence*, Susan Griffin develops a theory of the "pornographic mind" which, she claims, is the foundation of our culture and permeates every aspect of our lives:

> [T]he pornographic mind is a mind in which we all participate. It is the mind which dominates our culture. A mind which speaks to us through philosophy and literature, through religious doctrine and art, through film, through advertisement, in the commonest gestures, in our habits, through history and our ideas of history, and in the random acts of violence which surround our lives. (3)

According to Griffin, the development of Western culture and civilization is based on its separation from nature. Unlike Freud, who claimed that the conflict between nature and culture is inevitable and that the subjugation of nature is necessary for the development of culture (Griffin 128), Griffin argues that a unity between the two is possible and she refers to this wholeness as *eros*. Like Freud, however, she sees this drama played out on two levels: in a human being as a choice between body (id) and mind (ego, superego), and in our society as a choice between nature and culture. Griffin argues that our culture's decision to separate itself from nature was based on the fear of the power of nature. Hence, we believe that the subjugation of nature is necessary for our survival. However, it is impossible to suppress or master nature. Therefore, the scenario of subjugation is played out over

223 Sontag's article is not a feminist critique of pornography. Her argument is concerned with selected pornographic books as works of art.

and over again. Since woman is traditionally associated with nature, it is her body that becomes the site of the struggle. In addition, Griffin claims, the woman's body makes a heterosexual man aware of his own physicality and vulnerability. Therefore, he imagines himself to be in control of the female body and in control of nature as a result. According to Griffin, this fantasy of subjugation is realized in pornography by the objectification and humiliation of women. Pornography exaggerates the triumph of man (culture) over woman (nature) by stripping the female body of its spiritual dimension and by turning it into flesh. The alleged female inferiority is supposed to justify the degradation. Griffin writes:

> The image of woman as a void is a dominant theme of pornographic culture. A woman is less. She is less strong, less intelligent, less creative, less spiritual. She does not exist for herself. Rather, she is a shadow, whose existence depends on the real existence of men. She exists for men [...] Therefore the pornographic mind conceives of female sexuality as a kind of bottomless pit, an empty space which craves male presence, and which cannot exist without the male. (218)

As argued by Griffin, in a pornographic representation, woman cannot exist without a man. In addition, her humanity and individuality are erased. She becomes equated with her materiality. Her body is often fragmented and reduced to selected elements. She is associated with animals and perceived as a representative of a less valuable species. Her sexuality is believed to be dependent on men and is always the focus of representation. In her discussion of "the pornographic mind," however, Griffin argues that "the pornographic mind" manifests itself not only in sexism but also in all other instances of discrimination of particular social groups, such as anti-Semitism and racism. I decided to use the term "the pornographic imagination" in relation to Möbius' text to emphasize the specific nature of the gender discrimination he promotes. I also contend that *Über den physiologischen Schwachsinn des Weibes* approaches texts that are openly pornographic much more closely than many other cultural products that Griffin considers to be manifestations of "the pornographic mind." It includes all the above discussed characteristics of pornography without being explicitly sexual.

5.4 Möbius' Text as an Expression of Pornographic Imagination

The title of the text itself indicates that the pamphlet has a misogynistic character. Although Möbius tries to justify the use of the word "Schwachsinn," his explanation does not free the term of its pejorative meaning. "Schwachsinn" in conjunction with "Weib" creates a strong impression of spitefulness and subjective personal opinion. Möbius starts his text by defining what feeble-mindedness is. It is "das, was zwischen Blödsinn und normalem Verhalten liegt" (*Schwachsinn* 25).

However, he admits it is difficult to draw a line between feeble-mindedness and normal behavior. He further relates "Schwachsinn" to everyday experience and compares the above distinction to the difference between "gescheit und dumm" (*Schwachsinn* 25). He concludes: "In der Tat dürfte zwischen der Dummheit und den leichten Formen des Schwachsinns kein wesentlicher Unterschied sein" (*Schwachsinn* 25-26). He goes on to apply his distinction to human beings. Thus, he claims that it is possible to find a norm against which intellectual capacity can be measured. For Möbius, this norm is that of an adult white male. He asserts: "Das normale Verhalten des Kindes ist bei dem Erwachsenen pathologisch, das des Weibes bei dem Manne, das des Negers bei dem Europäer" (*Schwachsinn* 27). According to Möbius, there are several types of human beings and therefore one cannot talk about humans in general. Each of these types can be compared only to the members of the same group because all types differ significantly in their diverse qualities. After establishing the norm against which all people should be measured, Möbius characterizes the main object of his investigation, *das Weib*. He defines her as follows: "Körperlich genommen, ist [...] das Weib ein Mittelding zwischen Kind und Mann und geistig ist sie es, wenigstens in vielen Hinsichten, auch" (*Schwachsinn* 28). In addition, a woman (*das Weib*) is "während eines beträchtlichen Teiles seines Lebens als abnorm anzusehen" (*Schwachsinn* 45). Like Runge before him, Möbius situates women much lower on the ladder of evolutionary development than men, but he goes even further when he suggests that a woman can or should be defined against an animal.

It is precisely the comparison or even the identification of woman with animal that constitutes the main theme of Möbius' work and provides for the degrading and humiliating tone of the pamphlet. The basis of such an association is the opposition between "Gattungswesen" and "Individuum" (*Schwachsinn* 31). "Gattungswesen," of which the animal is the prime example, is at the very bottom of the evolutionary ladder and acts mainly upon instincts and impulses. As species develop into more complex forms, they acquire additional qualities. Developed cognitive abilities characterize the "Individuum" that rose to the top of the evolutionary ladder. In Möbius' claims, the animal is a point of reference from which he attempts to characterize women because a female is located much closer to an animal than to man on the evolutionary ladder. Möbius points out that also Lombroso "gern auf das Tierreich verweist" and "[Lombroso] betont, daß im ganzen Tierreiche die Intelligenz im umgekehrten Verhältnisse zur Fruchtbarkeit stehe" (*Schwachsinn* 41-42). Möbius is especially drawn to Rüdinger's research because Rüdinger argued that the brain of a Bavarian woman he examined represented a "tierähnlichen Typus" (Möbius, *Schwachsinn* 29).[224] In addition, Möbius postulates instincts and drives as guiding forces of a woman's behavior. While a man is defined by his reason, a woman is an instinctive creature: "Der Instinkt nun macht das Weib tierähnlich, unselbständig, sicher und heiter" (Möbius, *Schwachsinn* 34).

224 See also Thorson 13-14.

Some of Möbius' comparisons of woman to animal are explicit like those quoted above, others imply such an association. For example, he says: "Wäre das Weib nicht körperlich und geistig schwach, wäre es nicht in der Regel durch die Umstände unschädlich gemacht, so wäre es höchst gefährlich" (Möbius, *Schwachsinn* 35). This description is reminiscent of a domesticated wild animal that would be dangerous had it not been appropriately raised and controlled. A quite detailed description of female characteristics starts with the following statement: "*Wie die Tiere* seit undenklichen Zeiten immer dasselbe tun, so würde auch das menschliche Geschlecht, wenn es nur Weiber gäbe, in seinem Urzustande geblieben sein" (Möbius, *Schwachsinn* 34; emphasis added). Möbius develops this assertion as follows: "Mit dieser *Tierähnlichkeit* hängen sehr viele weibliche Eigentümlichkeiten zusammen" (*Schwachsinn* 34; emphasis added). They include: "Mangel eigenen Urteils" (34), "Enge des Gesichtskreises" (35), "Heftigkeit der Affekte" (35), "Unzulänglichkeit der Beherrschung" (35), and "Zanksucht und Schwatzhaftigkeit" (36) to name a few. In addition, women are "streng konservativ und hassen das Neue" (34), unable "das Gute vom Bösen [...] zu unterscheiden" (34), and "moralisch einseitig und defekt" (35). He further asserts: "Das Schwatzen gewährt dem Weibe unendliches Vergnügen, ist der eigentliche weibliche Sport. Vielleicht läßt sich das verstehen, wenn man an *die Übungsspiele der Tiere* denkt" (Möbius, *Schwachsinn* 36; emphasis added). Consequently, he also refers to the differences that allow one to distinguish between a woman and an animal: "Das menschliche Weib soll nicht nur Kinder gebären, sondern auch diese pflegen, da sie, im Gegensatze zu den Jungen der Tiere, soundso viele Jahre lang hilfebedürftig bleiben. *Diese Hilfebedürftigkeit der Kinder macht beim Menschen eine größere Differenzierung der Geschlechter nötig als bei den Tieren*" (Möbius, *Schwachsinn* 40). Möbius suggests, as mentioned above, that while women remained almost entirely at the same level of development as animals, men were able to develop into complete human beings. This stagnation of female development manifests itself primarily through the lack of cognitive abilities: "Das Weib ist nämlich nicht nur karger mit Geistesgaben versehen, als der Mann, sondern sie büßt sie auch viel rascher wieder ein" (Möbius, *Schwachsinn* 46). A significant part of the pamphlet is dedicated to the discussion of different types of cognitive abilities and skills. Möbius does not deny that women can think, but he argues that they are unable to think independently, critically, or creatively: "Verständnis und Gedächtnis sind bei vielen Weibern, soweit wie nicht besondere Talente in Frage kommen, durchaus nicht schlecht. [...] Dagegen ist [...] das Erfinden, Schaffen neuer Methoden, dem Weibe versagt" (*Schwachsinn* 36-37). To these defects he adds: "Mangel an Vermögen, zu kombinieren" (*Schwachsinn* 38), "das Fehlen selbständigen Denkens" (*Schwachsinn* 38), and "Mangel an Sachlichkeit" (*Schwachsinn* 38).

Like most of the opponents of higher education for women, Möbius connects intellect, physical appearance, and reproductive functions. This claim had already been discussed in the previous chapters, so I will only mention it briefly here. However, I will emphasize the points that are important for my discussion of the extremely misogynist character of this text. Möbius claims that because a woman is naturally animal-like, the development of her cognitive abilities would erase, at least partially, her animal nature which, in turn, would lead to a development of unnatural and abnormal characteristics. Talent, for example, is a pathological feature in a woman and has negative consequences for her femininity: "Ganz selten findet man ein wirkliches Talent, und dann pflegen auch andere Züge den geistigen Hermaphroditismus darzutun" (*Schwachsinn* 37-38). Möbius argues that an intellectual woman is a "Mann mit einem Uterus" (*Schwachsinn* 41). Hence, Möbius defines femininity based on intellectual and psychological, but not anatomical, qualities. As exemplified by this quotation, the uterus is not the female gender characteristic. Instead, the lack of talents and intellect becomes the marker of femininity.

Like most who made this argument, Möbius posits the deterioration in the female ability to reproduce as a consequence of intensive intellectual activity: "Offenbar ist das Urphänomen der Gegensatz zwischen Gehirntätigkeit und Fortpflanzung. Beide Funktionen sind eng verknüpft, aber je mehr die eine das Übergewicht erhält, um so mehr leidet die andere. [...] Ein wesentliches Kennzeichen dieser Form der Entartung ist die Verwischung der Geschlechtscharaktere: weibische Männer und männische Weiber" (*Schwachsinn* 44). Intellectual activity is "Misshandlung des weiblichen Gehirns" (*Schwachsinn* 44) and "[ü]bermäßige Gehirntätigkeit macht das Weib nicht nur verkehrt, sondern auch krank" (*Schwachsinn* 41). Möbius further argues that if a woman acquires any of the qualities that are traditionally considered male, she will lose both her physical appeal and her ability to reproduce: "Ließe es sich machen, daß die weiblichen Fähigkeiten den männlichen gleich entwickelt würden, so würden die Mutterorgane verkrümmern, und wir würden einen häßlichen und nutzlosen Zwitter vor uns haben" (*Schwachsinn* 41).[225] The terms "häßlich" and "nutzlos" are crucial not only for this passage, but also for the entire pamphlet because they indicate that a woman's entire role is to be a dependent subject of heterosexual male desires.

Responses to Möbius at the beginning of the twentieth century demonstrate that many intellectuals and activists read the pamphlet as a manifestation of the pornographic imagination. In many ways, their critiques resemble the analysis of pornography in contemporary radical feminist thought. Johanna Elberskirchen[226] emphasizes Möbius' focus on female sexuality in conjunction with objectifying descriptions and dehumanizing comparisons. She argues that most of the male physicians and scientists are not able to speak objectively about the "Woman Question" and feminism: "Sie stehen dem Weibe zu persönlich und zu materialistisch gegenüber und beurteilen es aus einer ganz schiefen und recht beschränkten Perspektive, jedenfalls von ganz unwissenschaftlichen Gesichtspunkten aus" (Elberskirchen 3). She implies that their subjective views are conditioned by sexual

225 Also qtd. in Thorson 15.

226 See also Thorson's analysis of Elberskirchen's response to Möbius 26.

urges. They perceive women exclusively as bodies and see therefore only their material dimensions. In addition, male physicians and scientists have been influenced and conditioned by tradition and culture. In spite of their education and scholarship, they are unable to distance themselves from "tausendjährigen Suggestionen" about women (Elberskirchen 4). These scientists and physicians are not able to view women as neutral patients but act upon their sexual urges and perceive their patients purely as sexual beings. She claims: "Tatsache ist, daß die Gelehrten gegenüber dem Weibe in ihrem Urteil zu sehr Mann und zu wenig oder gar nicht wissenschaftlich urteilender Mensch sind. Sie vergessen alle Wissenschaft, alle Empirie, alle wissenschaftlichen Erkenntnisse [...] wo sie über das Weib ein Urteil abgeben" (Elberskirchen 4). Elberskirchen argues that these scientists look at women and see only their material dimensions, their bodies, but do not perceive women as complete human beings. Hence, under the male scientific gaze the self and individuality of a woman are erased. She is reduced to a sexual being: "[S]ie sehen im Weibe nur *das Weib*, das Geschlechtswesen, am Weibe nur das Geschlecht und vor lauter Sexus sehen sie nicht das Menschliche, das Individuelle, das Ich im Weibe" (Elberskirchen 4). Elberskirchen's response clearly implies a pornographic imagination underlying Möbius' text as Möbius creates images in which women are depicted as sexual objects and equated with their bodies. The question of femininity is reduced to a discussion of female reproductive organs; hence, even the female body ceases to be a complex entity as it is fragmented in Möbius' text. Exactly as in pornography, woman is equated with her sexual organs or secondary sexual characteristics, her individuality is erased, and she does not have any purpose of existence besides that of providing pleasure to men. Elberskirchen develops her argument as follows:

> Sie [die Gelehrten] messen das Weib mit dem Maßstabe des Sexus und ordnen das Gehirn des Weibes, entgegen den einfachsten anatomischen, physiologischen Tatsachen seinem Sexualorgan unter, die Persönlichkeit des Weibes seiner geschlechtlichen Eigentümlichkeit, die doch nur ein Bruchteil der Persönlichkeit ist, und behaupten, die Persönlichkeit, das Ich des Weibes werde in seinem wesentlichen Bestande durch seine geschlechtliche Eigentümlichkeit bestimmt und sei davon vollständig abhängig! (4-5)

In the discourses produced by scientists and physicians, female individuality and intellect are equated with sexuality. Woman does not have a personality that transcends the sexual. In her text, Elberskirchen contests such a representation and emphasizes the personality, character, and self of women, thus neutralizing the image Möbius creates. What Möbius sees as an inherent normal female quality, Elberskirchen defines as pathological: "Es ist stets ein Symptom der Entartung, wenn eine der Komponenten eine führende Rolle im Organismus übernimmt und mehr Kräfte aufsaugt, als ihr ursprünglich zukommen" (6). She claims that women's sexuality shapes female personality only to a certain degree and cannot be equated with woman herself, as Möbius suggests: "Die geschlechtliche Eigentümlichkeit ist [...] ein Teil des weiblichen Menschen und gibt seiner geschlechtlichen Persönlichkeit eine ganz bestimmte Färbung, sie ist aber niemals dieser weibliche Mensch selbst und wirkt niemals bestimmend auf die menschliche Persönlichkeit des Weibes, auf den Charakter" (Elberskirchen 8).

Elberskirchen seems to address the ideology underlying Möbius' text in terms of the pornographic imagination in a much more obvious and detailed way than other women responding to the pamphlet. However, she is not the only one who appears to make such a connection. For example, Asmus agrees that *Über den physiologischen Schwachsinn des Weibes* publicly humiliates women by focusing on their sexuality. She states: "Das ist kein wissenschaftliches, sachliches Untersuchen, das ist ein Daraufloswüten, das den ehrwürdigen Gegenstand abscheulich macht" (Asmus 239). Asmus also maintains that Möbius' book evokes "das peinliche Gefühl gegen ein unlogisches Werk [...], [...] gegenüber einem unklaren Prinzip" (232). Similarly, Bülow emphasizes the derogatory and demeaning portrayal of women. According to her, Möbius' text created "von dem gesunden, naturgemäßen Weibe und seiner Stellung ein [...] abstoßendes Bild" (Bülow, "Schwachsinn" 17).

Dohm implies that Möbius' text is a personal, sexually tainted vengeance fantasy parading as a scientific text. She claims that Möbius could not have acquired knowledge about women in an empirical way, because a woman as created by his text does not exist and is only a male fantasy, an imaginary formation of the text:

> Wie erwerben deutsche gelehrte Herren à la Möbius ihre Kenntnis der Frauennatur? Auf empirischem Wege kaum. So trefflich ethisch beschlagene Wissenschaftler wie er haben sich voraussichtlich als Jünglinge von der Hefe des Frauentums fern gehalten, nicht wie Schopenhauer haben sie sich aus dem Verkehr mit Dirnen ihre Anschauungen über das Weib gebildet. [...] Daß ein Möbius nach der Verheiratung noch Verlangen getragen haben sollte, mit dem schwachsinnigen Geschlecht einen lebhaften geistigen Verkehr zu pflegen, ist mehr als unwahrscheinlich. [...] Wahrscheinlich ist er [Möbius] gar nicht verheiratet, oder er hat eine ungeheuer kluge Frau, was ihn fürchterlich ärgert, und seine Schrift ist nichts als eine Rache, die er an ihr nimmt. (Dohm, "Randglossen" 36)

Dohm speculates that Möbius' frustration and unfulfilled personal life were the main motives for writing the pamphlet. As a matter of fact, Möbius' biography confirms her assumptions. According to Ernst Jentsch, Möbius married in 1879 but "[d]ie Ehe blieb kinderlos, und die Frau starb 1902, nachdem sie in den letzten Jahren von ihm getrennt gelebt hatte, ohne daß die Ehe gerichtlich geschieden war" (6). Jentsch further informs the reader that Möbius did not have any friends and lead a completely withdrawn and secluded life (6). According to Dohm, *Über den physiologischen Schwachsinn des Weibes* is a personal revenge-fantasy that allows Möbius to see women as subordinated, not threatening, and unequal to men. Dohm further points out that Möbius discusses femininity through the prism of sexual fantasies: "Die Tierähnlichkeit macht sie [die Frau] bewundernswert? Wir nehmen Acht von diesem Bekenntnis. Dafür kann man aber doch das Weib nicht strafen (durch Entziehung der Geistesnahrung), daß der Mann in ihr das Tier so liebt. Wie recht hatte Helene Böhlau, ihren letzten Roman 'Halbtier' zu nennen, oder wäre 'Ganztier' noch passender gewesen?" (Dohm, "Randglossen" 19). As indicated by Dohm, Möbius creates a representation of women that, like pornography aimed at heterosexual men, conforms to the male fantasies but not to the demands or wishes of women themselves.

In summary, women's responses to Möbius' text at the beginning of the twentieth century demonstrate that *Über den physiologischen Schwachsinn des Weibes* constructs an image of femininity that is comfortable and unthreatening to men, gives all women the same instrumental value, and elevates the male to a superior status. In light of these reactions, the pamphlet reveals itself as a display of the alleged male superiority that is not questioned or undermined, where woman becomes a dependent object of male power and is reduced to her materiality. It further erases woman's intellectual and spiritual dimensions as it equates her with the body. Seen from this perspective, Möbius' pamphlet is not just an ephemeral publication with a provocative title. It is rather a manifestation of patriarchal ideology taken to its extreme.

5.5 From Nature to Culture: Progress of Civilization

Besides the scientific and artistic obsession with sexual differences and gender distinctions between men and women, discussions about progress and civilization as well as about the relationship of nature and culture constituted a quite popular topic in science and philosophy at the turn of the twentieth century. Schmersahl emphasized, for example, "das Bestreben von Sexualwissenschaftlern [...] kulturhistorische Theorien und Themen in das Feld der Medizin zu integrieren und naturwissenschaftlich zu begründen" (112). Many scientists combined the theory of evolution with claims about culture and civilization, especially while discussing questions of sex and gender. As a result of such unifying approaches encompassing a broad range of disciplines, as Schmersahl argues, "[d]ie entwicklungsgeschichtliche Theorie, nach der Zivilisation und Fortschritt mit einer hohen Differenzierung der Geschlechter und einer monogamen Heterosexualität korrespondierten, wurde damit zum Naturgesetz erhoben" (Schmersahl 112). As already noted,[227] many scientists shared a quite pessimistic view of modern cultural

227 See footnote 218.

developments and saw the appearance of "Mannweiber" as a reflection of civilization gone the wrong way. Women publicly displaying "male characteristics," demanding access to the spheres reserved exclusively for men, and refusing to confine themselves to the private realm negated the principle of difference between men and women that was believed to be a sign of progress and evolutionary development. By collapsing "male" and "female" qualities into one, they exemplified, according to the scientific view of the time, biological and cultural degeneration of the whole Western civilization.[228]

The opposition of nature, associated with women, and culture, associated with men, is one of the fundamental dichotomies evoked by the opponents of women's emancipation. Möbius attempts to uphold this division and argues that culture should further enhance distinctions (such as the differences between men and women) that were, according to him, created by nature. In the context of *Über den physiologischen Schwachsinn des Weibes*, this means maintaining the underprivileged position of women in society. Olberg, Dohm, Bülow, Gumplowicz, and Elberskirchen respond to his claims in four different ways. Olberg analyzes the development of human civilization in terms of its progress from the state of nature to the state of culture and sees women's emancipation as one of the most advanced developments within society. According to her, the subjugation of women (the weaker) might have been a natural state, but it is not the cultural state. Hence, she glorifies culture as a means to achieve the equality of women. In so doing, she also erases the opposition between nature/woman and culture/man. Unlike Olberg, Dohm recognizes that there are many oppressive and therefore regressive elements in the cultural development, one of them being the subjugation of women. Gender inequality and oppression of women are creations of culture/civilization and need to be recognized as such. Similar to Dohm, Bülow sets up the distinction between raw nature and civilization. The main task of human culture is to correct injustices created by nature, for example, the inequality of the sexes. Gumplowicz points out that people have very different functions and obligations in the natural and the cultural states and therefore both types of conditions create different types of people. Consequently gender relations are different. Hence, one cannot impose gender relations of the natural state onto the cultural state. Elberskirchen participates in the debate about culture and civilization by addressing the connection between sexuality and culture.[229]

---

228 See also Schmersahl 39-113 and her discussion of Möbius in this context 325-326. Schmersahl also points out that there also were intellectuals who believed the opposite, claiming that "[die] Angleichung der Geschlechter" was a sign of progress (340). These individuals "rekrutierten sich [...] aus dem Lager derjenigen Frauen, die sich in die hitzige Debatte um die Geschlechter mischten, und aus dem Umfeld von Magnus Hirschfeld" (340).

229 Weiershausen demonstrated that the discussion about culture, civilization, and nature in the context of women's emancipation spilled over into literary works of the time. Erwin Guido Kolbenheyer's novel *Montsalvasch* is a case in point. For more details, see Weiershausen 167-171; 175-178; 179-182. As Weiershausen points out, "culture" and "civilization" have

In *Das Weib und der Intellectualismus,* Olberg responds to Möbius' pamphlet by addressing the opposition between nature and culture/civilization. She points out that it is impossible to address the "Woman Question" without investigating the broader worldview that underlies this issue. According to Olberg, the question of women's intellectual development is embedded in the distinction between nature and culture/civilization. Therefore she deems it necessary to offer an analysis of culture, society, and the development of civilization as a background against which Mobius' claims can be discussed.

Olberg emphasizes that the opponents of women's intellectual development are deluded by a kind of fantasy in which they situate women as close to the "state of nature" as possible. In order to realize this vision, they try to exclude women from participation in the achievements of civilization and argue that such exclusion is not only natural but also necessary for the good of the community. They usually claim that a woman's intellectual pursuit is unnatural and would lead to societal degeneration. These arguments constitute the main core of all arguments trying to dismiss the "Woman Question" and result in a back-to-nature-postulate that is impossible to fulfill as people have already significantly progressed and this development cannot be reversed. Olberg reminds her readers that cultural advancements were necessitated by external circumstances and human needs: "an der Wiege der Cultur [hat] die unerbittliche Notwendigkeit der Selbsterhaltung gestanden" (29). Civilization developed as a means to improve people's lives and is an expression of the drive to preserve the species and make individual survival possible. Therefore, any attempt to reverse these changes is not only deemed to be unsuccessful, but also unreasonable.

Human intellect has been the driving force behind the development of culture and it is impossible to separate the two. Möbius, however, perceives intellectual development in women as something that actually causes a person and civilization to deteriorate:

> Auf diesem Boden steht auch Professor Moebius, der [...] die Meinung ausspricht, dass die Bildung ihre Jünger ohne Erbarmen umbringt, indem sie deren Familien auf den Aussterbeetat setzt [...], dass die Wochenbetten um so schlechter, die Milchabsonderung um so geringer, die Weiber um so untauglicher werden, je besser die Schulen sind [...], und der deshalb annimmt, dass es im Interessen der Menschheit liege, durch die Natürlichkeit des Weibes der Gehirncultur ein Gegengewicht zu schaffen. (Olberg 31)

According to Olberg, mankind evolves through cultural development and one cannot arbitrarily exclude one group (women) from this process. The question of women's intellectual development did not arise in a vacuum, but became an

for Kolbenheyer two different meanings. Writers discussed in this section use "culture" and "civilization" as synonyms.

integral component of modern culture. Women are part of civilization and of cultural development to the same degree as men: "Was darzuthun ist, ist nicht das Recht des Weibes auf geistige Entfaltung schlechthin, sondern in einem gegebenen culturellen Milieu, dessen Entwicklung in einer gegebenen Richtung als angestrebt vorausgesetzt wird" (Olberg 21). According to Olberg, women's demands for education and intellectual development are inevitable consequences of a broader cultural development, namely modernity. Hence "das moderne Streben des Weibes" (Olberg 87) is a modern postulate. In other words, Olberg defines modernity by equating it with the emancipation of women.

The further people progress from the "state of nature" the more they rely on their intellect and the more they try to expand their cognitive functions. Therefore women's struggle for equality is a sign of cultural progress and not of degeneration. In addition, Olberg points out that the development of culture is paralleled by the transformation of a biological human being into a social human being. Among other developments that are specific to this evolution, Olberg stresses that the human brain undergoes changes: "die langsame structurelle Verfeinerung und Vermehrung des Volumens im Gehirn des Culturmenschen" (35). Women are obviously not excluded from these evolutionary transformations and should be given an opportunity to use their intellect to its fullest potential.

Olberg responds to the programmatic aspect of Möbius' pamphlet and points out that his call to reverse women's emancipation can be equated with an attempt to dismiss all achievements of civilization and cultural progress:

> Die Gegner der Frauenfrage pflegen ihre Abneigung gegen die moderne Cultur nur gelegentlich einzuflechten [...]. [...] Wens nach dem Mittelalter oder meinetwegen nach vorsintflutlichen Perioden zurückzieht, wer meint, die Culturmenschheit gehe einen falschen Weg, der sage es offen und gehe von diesem Standpunkt aus in seiner Kritik der Frauenfrage [...]. (Olberg 40)

For Olberg, one cannot reverse emancipatory developments without reversing the progress of mankind. Möbius does not recognize or does not want to recognize this connection and fantasizes, according to Olberg, about retaining "Das Weib [...] als 'Stück Natur' inmitten der modernen [...] Welt" (60). She sees Möbius' postulate as a manifestation of the Rousseauian nostalgia with a strong misogynist twist, as only women are supposed to revert back to nature while men enjoy cultural and technological advancements. So far, Olberg argues, the development of culture and civilization had made life easier for men:

> Die menschliche Naturbeherrschung, die die Gewinnung der Existenzmittel erleichtert und Gefahren ausschaltet, entlastet den Mann als Ernährer und bietet die Möglichkeit, die Frau als Gebärerin und Pflegerin der Nachkommenschaft zu entlasten. [...] Ein Rückblick

> auf die Geschichte zeigt uns, dass die Entlastung des Mannes viel früher einsetzt, als die des Weibes. (41)

Due to their privileged position in society, men were able to use the advantages of cultural progress much earlier than women. Women, too, are entitled to the advantages that civilization created, but the opponents of women's emancipation attempt to impede this development: "Von den Gegnern der Frauenbewegung wird auf diesen 'Naturzustand' hingewiesen, als auf das Urbild der weiblichen Function. Diese Auffassung der menschlichen Fortpflanzung stellt das Weib ausserhalb des Culturgebietes, will ihm keine Entlastung in seinem Dienste der Art zuerkennen" (Olberg 43). Olberg points out that woman is as much a part of culture as man. This fact cannot be changed by either Möbius or any other opponent of women's emancipation even if he strongly believes in his peculiar vision.

As part of her argument about nature, progress, and civilization, Olberg discusses the connection between intellectual development and female fertility at length and contends that there is indeed a close relationship between the two. Olberg agrees with Möbius that a higher level of intellectual or cultural development can lead to a reduced birth rate, but according to her, since the mortality rate declines simultaneously, both developments balance each other out: "Wenn eine Gesellschaft die Zahl der Todesursachen vermindert, so lässt sie eine Verminderung der Fruchtbarkeit zu" (Olberg 42). It is natural that if a species improves its survival skills, its fertility declines (Olberg 43). Consequently, as the human race develops and progresses, there is no need for a high fertility rate: "Die ungeheure Fruchtbarkeit der niederen Tiere [...] geht dem höheren Tiere unfehlbar verloren" (Olberg 44). In her discussion of fertility and culture, Olberg emphasizes the difference between "leiblicher und seelischer Fruchtbarkeit" as well as the difference between "der Mutterschaft als animalischer und der Mutterschaft als menschlicher Function" (51). According to her, since Möbius does not make this distinction at all, he cannot be taken seriously. Physical motherhood, or, in other words, the ability to give birth is a feature of all female organisms. But the most important difference between a human being and an animal is the woman's ability to educate and rear children within the social context. Olberg emphasizes again that as culture and civilization progressed, women developed to perceive motherhood less as a physiological and more as an intellectual and spiritual task:

> Das sociale Ergebnis ist ein erhöhter Schutz des heranwachsenden Lebens vor der Ungunst der äusseren Bedingungen, das individuelle eine verminderte Ausgabe an plastischer Energie, eine Durchdringung der Mütterlichkeit mit intellectuellen Elementen, ein Einbeziehen des Weibes in das geistige Leben der Gesellschaft, auf der einen Seite, weil die Mutterschaft von der animalischen Function mehr zur menschlichen wird und dem Kinde in seinem psychischen Entfaltungs- und Anpassungsprocess zur Seite steht, auf der anderen

> Seite, weil die verminderte Geburtenzahl einen Ueberschuss lässt, der zwar als erhöhte Sorgfalt der Nachkommenschaft wieder zugewandt wird, mit der fortschreitenden Entwicklung der öffentlichen Gesundheitspflege, der Verteilung der heute zusammengepferchten Bevölkerungsmassen, der Schaffung eines den Bedürfnissen des heranwachsenden Geschlechtes angemessenen Milieus der intellectuellen Ausbildung des Weibes zugewendet werden kann. (58)

Olberg argues that the lower mortality rate in connection with cultural and technological developments could (and should) be used to propose exactly the opposite of what Möbius calls for, that is, a reduced birth rate and women's intellectual development: "Im Gegensatz zu denen, die von der Notwendigkeit einer hohen Fruchtbarkeit ausgehen, um für das Weib Ausschluss aus der Sphäre der intellectuellen Cultur zu fordern, könnte man von der Reduction der Fruchtbarkeit als Postulat ausgehen, um zur Forderung intellectueller Thätigkeit des Weibes zu kommen" (62). Olberg emphasizes that due to technological and cultural advancements, women do not have to devote as much time to their children and can use the surplus of energy for themselves. Hence, she dismisses Möbius' appeal to recognize and maintain female feeble-mindedness as "Mittel zur Erhaltung einer hohen Fruchtbarkeit" (Olberg 61).

In her critique of Möbius, Olberg points out that he holds onto the traditionally established split between nature and culture and does not recognize that this division should be bridged as there is no contradiction between women's demands for intellectual attainment and the good of society: "Ein Antagonismus zwischen dem Wohle der Art und dem des Individuums ist hier so recht bei den Haaren herbeigezogen worden. In Wirklichkeit besteht eine innige Solidarität der Interessen" (Olberg 88). Instead of presenting an opposition between nature and culture, between woman and man, Olberg proposes a dialectical union of the two:

> Die von transcendentalen Werturteilen imprägnierte Auffassung, nach der der Mensch vom Intellect nach "oben" und von den Trieben nach "unten" gezerrt wird, hat fast allen Boden verloren. Die gesunde Intelligenz wendet sich nicht gegen die gesunden Forderungen des Trieblebens oder es kommt doch nur zu leichten oder vorübergehenden Conflicten, bei denen im Grunde nicht Erkenntnis gegen das Gefühl steht, sondern der sociale Mensch gegen den biologischen. (105)

Like Olberg, Dohm discusses the opposition between nature and culture, but whereas Olberg emphasizes the liberating aspect of cultural development, Dohm stresses subjugation and inequality as created and supported by customs and traditions inherent in every civilization. According to her, the tale about female feeble-mindedness is part of this oppressive tradition. Although Möbius claims that it is natural, in reality it is a cultural construction. Möbius understands customs and traditions as an extension of nature and a support of only what was created by nature, while Dohm sees them as an opposition of nature: "Die Sitte wäre immer der Ausdruck des von der Natur gewollten gewesen? Die Sitten nicht ein Spiegel des Kulturzustandes der Zeit? Und nicht einmal das, oft sind sie nur ein Spiegel vergangener Kulturzustände" ("Randglossen" 19). For Möbius, according to Dohm, a woman is a fixed and unchanging entity that does not undergo evolutionary transformations. Möbius asserts "die Stabilität der Sitte" ("Randglossen" 19) and talks about "die Beschaffenheit des Weibes [...] zu allen Zeiten und in allen Völkern" (qtd. in Dohm, "Randglossen" 19). According to Dohm, customs and cultures developed as a result of the subjugation of nature and they are constantly changing. For Möbius, on the other hand, they are stable entities without evolutionary progress. Dohm argues that, depending on the community, customs and traditions were established either for the good of the people upon mutual agreement or to the advantage of the ruling group. As time passed, these traditions and customs became self-evident, their origins were forgotten, and people failed to remember that they were socially constructed and perceived them as created by nature ("Randglossen" 19). Dohm further questions the validity of the oppressive traditions and practices and suggests that they should be changed if they no longer serve people. She suggests that it is our obligation to question social practices and try to find the source and motivation behind traditions that seem so natural to people like Möbius. The longer a tradition exists the more appropriate it is to question its validity ("Randglossen" 19).

Since social practices, beliefs, and traditions were invented by people, they are changeable. Not only is it possible to change them, but they also should be changed when they do not serve people any more. As the human race progresses, it requires new and different norms and rules of behavior. Such changes are then signs of progress and not degeneration. "Die Stabilität der Sitte" (Dohm, "Randglossen" 19) that Möbius proclaims, indicates, according to Dohm, a lack of progress. As human knowledge and understanding change and develop, customs have to be changed as well in order to match the progress.

Dohm elaborates on her assertions by stressing the constructedness of categories such as class and gender. As the perception of reality changes, social practices and customs change as well. Once the understanding of these categories changes, then the position of people does too: "Die Tschandalas, die Parias, wurden durch Jahrtausende als tierische Geschöpfe von jedem Menschenrecht ausgeschlossen. Und die Sklaverei, die selbst dem edelsten Volke des Altertums als eine Naturnotwendigkeit galt [...]? [...] seit wie lange gilt denn nach Sitte und Herkommen der bürgerliche als ein dem Adel gleichberechtigter Staatsangehöriger?" (Dohm, "Randglossen" 19). She further states that these categories and notions are socially constructed and arbitrary: "Sprach nicht noch Metternich das freche Wort: 'Der Mensch fängt erst mit dem Baron an.' Und neulich hörte ich sogar von einem lieben, ehrwürdigen Professor der Mathematik, daß der zivilisierte

Menach erst mit dem Mathematiker anfinge. Der Herr Möbius [...] übertrumpft sie: Der Mensch fängt erst mit dem Manne an, und bei der Frau hört er auf" (Dohm, "Randglossen" 19).

Taking issue with traditional assumptions that culture should uphold the differences created by nature, Bülow's argument centers on human dignity as a cultural and not natural construct. Like Möbius, Bülow sets up a strong opposition between nature and culture, but her terms of opposition are very different. She juxtaposes the raw rules of nature, for example, survival of the fittest, with the laws established by people that were created to protect the weaker from the stronger. These laws uphold human dignity. Therefore, averting the negative impact of nature is one of the main tasks of culture and civilization:

> Obwohl die Natur den Schwächeren durch den Stärkeren gewürgt haben will, wollen wir Das nicht, sondern wir setzen dem Naturrecht des Stärkeren ein anderes, menschliches Recht entgegen, das uns vornehmer erscheint. Hier würde allerdings bereits die Abwendung von der Natur beginnen, die jede Kultur mit sich bringt als den Todeskeim. Wiederum ist aber alle Fortentwicklung Naturgesetz, so daß auch die scheinbare Abkehr von der Natur noch durch die Natur selbst und in ihr sich als Nothwendigkeit vollzieht. (Bülow, "Schwachsinn" 15)

A transition from the laws of nature to the laws created by people is a sign of progress. But at the same time, evolution and progress are laws of nature. Hence, overcoming nature is a law given by nature. According to Bülow, nature is brutal and culture is noble. Because love of justice is an inborn quality of mankind, a shift from nature to culture is inevitable.

> Gerechtigkeitliebe [sic] ist eine Anlage des Menschen, die zwar leicht verkrüppeln und verkrümmen kann, die ihn aber immer nöthigen wird, den Brutalitäten der Natur ein eigenes, verfeinertes, veredeltes Wollen entgegenzusetzen. Ja, der Mensch wird selbst dann noch dem eigenen Gerechtigkeitgefühl [sic] folgen müssen, wenn er selbst darüber zu Grunde gehen sollte. Wir müßten aus unserem eigenen Gefühl heraus die Natur korrigieren, wenn sie wirklich so grausam ungerecht und roh am Weibe gehandelt hätte, wie Möbius annimmt. Und zwar unter allen Umständen, es möge daraus werden, was wolle. Eben so wenig wie wir uns heute auf Kosten von Sklaven bereichern wollen, können wir den männlichen Theil unserer Rasse dadurch stärken wollen, daß wir die weibliche Hälfte ihrem Kulturverlangen zum Trotz auf mögliche Thierstufe herabdrücken. (Bülow, "Schwachsinn" 15-16)

Gumplowicz addresses the distinction between nature and culture in relation to motherhood. Unlike motherhood in the state of nature that Möbius advocates for women, motherhood in the state of culture/civilization requires the mother's education and knowledge: "Kehren wir die Frage erst einmal um: inwieweit kann eine Frau – nicht im Urwald, sondern innerhalb der Culturmenschheit – ihren Mutterpflichten genügen ohne geistige Arbeit?" (Gumplowicz 910). He argues that the separation of motherhood and intellect is not only undesirable, but also not possible in the state to which people have evolved. Mothers have to be educated in order to rear children responsibly. Gumplowicz argues that the turn of the twentieth century is marked by a profound change that brings about a new culture and new codes of behavior. Therefore we need a new mother who can rear children who will be prepared to live in this new world:

> Eine Tradition mechanisch weitergeben, das mag auch der frommen Einfalt gelingen; aber in einer revolutionären Zeit, wie die unsere, die auf allen Lebensgebieten die alten Normen unbrauchbar macht, der Jugend ratend und helfend zur Seite stehen bei dem schwierigen Werke des Sicheinlebens in eine werdende neue Cultur, eine Cultur mit neuen Lebenszielen und neuer Sittlichkeit – wenn die fromme Einfalt vor diese Aufgabe gestellt wird, richtet sie greuliches Unheil an. (Gumplowicz 911)

Like Gumplowicz and the other authors responding to Möbius, Asmus emphasizes that the cultural development cannot be reversed by Möbius. According to her, Möbius' text is "[eine] rückwärts-kommandierende Abhandlung" (Asmus 235). She asks: "In welcher Welt lebt denn dieser Herr? Sieht und hört er denn nicht, was vorgeht? Das Milieu, in dem er lebt, und über das hinaus seine Interessen nicht zu gehen scheinen, ist unserem Heute ein fremdes" (Asmus 237).

Elberskirchen published *Feminismus und Wissenschaft*, in which she addressed the connection between sexuality and culture, as a response to Möbius in 1903. Hence, like the authors discussed above, Elberskirchen also participates in the debate about culture and civilization. She contends that the primary sign of civilization and cultural developments is the subordination of the sexual to the spiritual and cognitive dimensions. With this claim, she directly opposes Möbius, for whom a subordination of female sexuality to the cognitive sphere is a sign of degeneration. Thus, Elberskirchen denies that female sexuality has a profound influence on women's lives and behavior and that it determines all other spheres. Similarly, Elberskirchen reverses Möbius' causal explanation for the alleged lack of female intellect and argues that it is not the sexual organs that dominate and determine all other organs and functions. On the contrary, according to her, the spirit ("Geist") determines all other qualities in both men and women: "Die Voraussetzung des organisierten Lebens ist das organisierte Prinzip, die Kraft, der Geist. Dieses Prinzip ordnet sich im Haushalte des Organismus alles unter, alle

Organe, auch den Sexus" (Elberskirchen 6). Hence, Möbius overestimates the role of female sexuality in the development of a woman's personality and misinterprets its connection to other physiological functions: "Der Sexus [...] gibt niemals der Individualität das Gepräge, sondern er vernichtet sie, sobald er im Individuum zur Herrschaft gelangt und ihr das Gepräge aufdrücken will. Oder präziser gesagt, der Organismus ist schon im Zerfall, wenn der Sexus das Gepräge aufdrücken kann" (Elberskirchen 7). The dominance of the sexual sphere that Möbius postulates is not a normal or natural state, but rather a pathological feature and sign of degeneration: "Die Herrschaft des Sexus ist stets ein Zeichen des Niedergangs. Das Individuum, dessen Sexus im Haushalte seines Organismus sozusagen eine führende bestimmende Rolle spielt, ist in der Entartung begriffen" (Elberskirchen 6). Whereas for Möbius a developed female intellect is a sign of degeneration, for Elberskirchen the degeneration is represented by the dominance of the sexual sphere. She associates sexuality (as defined by Möbius) with destruction. Sexuality that is tamed by culture, spirit, and intellect is a sign of cultural development.

5.6 Feminist Interpretation of Biological Data

The most striking aspect of *Feminismus und Wissenschaft* is Elberskirchen's reading of the male and female bodies as well as her feminist re-interpretation of biological data. While the authors discussed earlier in this chapter emphasized the role of culture and civilization in both subordination and emancipation of women, Elberskirchen focuses primarily on biology. Her interpretation of biological data and the conclusions she draws are completely different from the mainstream cultural perception of the time and support her plea for gender equality.

Elberskirchen postulates that male and female sexual organs are identical in the very beginning of their development: "[E]s gibt in der Anlage kein prinzipiell männliches und prinzipiell weibliches Geschlecht. Die sexuelle Uranlage ist bei beiden Geschlechtern ein und dieselbe" (8). This statement has, of course, profound consequences for Elberskirchen's view of the sexes and gender relations; she makes it impossible to derive so-called male and female personality traits from the respective sexual organs. Hence, she disagrees with Möbius' assumption that the sexes are naturally different and that there are specific gender characteristics. According to her, "[w]ir finden alle Charaktereigenschaften unterschiedslos auf Mann und Weib verteilt" (Elberskirchen 8).

Elberskirchen demonstrates that the rudimentary basis of sexual organs is the same in men and women at conception. The elements that are different, male and female genitals, are secondary organs. The primary organs, the gonads, are identical in men and women. Thus, Elberskirchen differentiates between secondary sexual organs (external genitals) and primary sexual organs (internal gonads). The gonads, not the genitals, are the main organ and they are always unisexual. Elberskirchen writes:

> Mann und Weib haben [...] genau dieselben Geschlechtsorgane in der Anlage. Später erst tritt eine geschlechtliche Differenzierung ein in der Weise, daß sich beim Weibe bezw. beim Manne die spezifisch weiblichen bezw. spezifisch männlichen Organe entwickeln, während die spezifisch männlichen bezw. weiblichen in der Norm, in der Entwicklung stehen bleiben oder sich zurückbilden. So z.B. die Gebärmutter des Weibes, die beim Manne allerdings sich nicht weiter entwickelt, aber bei ihm als "uterus masculinus" erhalten ist. Der Mann besitzt also auch eine Gebärmutter! Diese Organe nun, die sich beim Manne bezw. beim Weibe entwickeln, während sie bei dem anderen Geschlecht nicht entwickelt werden, sind sämtlich *Hülfsorgane*, nicht das Hauptorgan, das eigentliche prinzipielle Geschlechtsorgan selbst, sie haben mithin keine prinzipielle Bedeutung. Bedeutung hat nur das Hauptorgan: die Sexual- oder Keimdrüse. [...] Die Keimdrüse nun, also das Wesentliche des männlichen und weiblichen Sexualapparates, ist in der Anlage *einheitlich, unisexuell, nicht bisexuell.* Es gibt in der Anlage keine spezifisch männliche und spezifisch weibliche Sexualdrüse, die sich wie die Hülfsorgane nur beim Weibe bezw. beim Manne entwickelt und beim anderen Geschlecht rudimentär bleibt oder sich zurückbildet. Die Keimdrüse ist das, und zwar das einzige Organ der Sexualanlage, das sich bei Mann und Weib entwickelt, das bei beiden Geschlechtern ein und dasselbe ist und bleibt und bei beiden Geschlechtern in Funktion tritt und nicht wie die Hülfsorgane nur beim Weibe bezw. beim Manne sich entwickelt und funktioniert. (9-11)

Elberskirchen's is the first substantial feminist effort to intervene in traditional science as she re-interprets biological and anatomical data. Her interpretation supports an absolute equality of men and women because, according to her, the sexes are essentially the same. Because most of the accounts about female inferiority derive from the reading of male and female sexual organs as principally and essentially different, Elberskirchen's re-interpretation of anatomical structures makes such claims about inequality and difference impossible: "[D]as Weib [steht] dem Manne an geistigen und körperlichen Kräften qualitativ und quantitativ gleich [...]. Der Mann stammt vom Weibe und Manne, auch das Weib. Beide sind als Resultanten der gleichen Komponenten, der gleichen Kräfte – wie ist ein qualitativer und quantitativer Unterschied denkbar – wie möglich?" (13). In addition, she claims, sexuality constitutes only one of many human functions and does not determine other qualities in human beings. Hence, a woman cannot be reduced to her sexuality:

> Die Natur kennt bezüglich des Weibes "kein nur." Sie behandelt das Geschlecht bei Weib und Mann als eine Eigenschaft, die sie, wie die

> vielen anderen Eigenschaften des Individuums, mögen sie nun seelischer, intellektueller oder körperlicher Natur sein, nach ihrem urewigen Gesetz der lebendigen Zahl, der philosophischen Mathematik sich vererben läßt, ohne ihr eine dominierende oder gar bestimmende Stellung im Organismus des Individuums zuzuerkennen. (Elberskirchen 13-14)

Women, for ages, have been reduced to their sexuality because they were defined by men. Such representation and perception is only "das Produkt tausendjähriger krankhafter Suggestionen und tausendjähriger Unterdrückung des Weibes [...] das Produkt einer tausendjährigen Herrschaft des männlichen Sexus über das Weib" (Elberskirchen 14).

Elberskirchen accentuates the devastating effects that the patriarchal power structure had on women which resulted in "eine körperliche, moralische und geistige Verkrüppelung des Weibes, eine Verkrüppelung seiner Persönlichkeit" (14). Women are not inferior to men by nature, but were forced into subordination and dependency due to male dominance:

> Das sind Kräfte, die von außen her mit Gewalt in die Entwicklung des Weibes eingreifen, diese Entwicklung hemmen, dem Weibe Kräfte rauben und so das Weib entwerten. Das ist die Ursache der relativen geistigen, moralischen und körperlichen Rückständigkeit des Weibes, diese äußere Vergewaltigung, nicht aber eine dem Weibe immanente, in seiner Anlage begründete und durch seine Geschlechtseigenschaft gegebene Inferiorität. Nach der ganzen sozialen und persönlichen Stellung von Mann und Weib zueinander kann diese entwertende Kraft ihre Wurzeln nur in dem sexuellen Verhältnis von Mann und Weib, in der Herrschaft des männlichen Sexus über das Weib haben. (Elberskirchen 14-15)

In *Über den physiologischen Schwachsinn des Weibes*, Möbius defines female sexuality as a force that is destructive primarily for women themselves and also for men, if left uncontrolled. Elberskirchen contests this theory by portraying male sexuality as destructive for women. It is not an internal and inborn force that incapacitates women, but rather it is an external factor: male sexual dominance. Elberskirchen uses the language of physical and sexual violence to depict the relationship between the sexes over the course of history. Her choice of words such as "Gewalt," "von außen hin eingreifen," "Kräfte rauben," "entwerten," "Vergewaltigung," "entwertende Kraft," reflects her understanding of woman's powerless position in society. Möbius sees this position as a natural consequence of female feeble-mindedness while Elberskirchen shows this hierarchical arrangement in a different light. She reads the subjugation of women as a consequence of male (hetero) sexual drive and dominance. Thus, she depicts the social history of gender relationships as a rape perpetrated on women.

The paragraph quoted above also illuminates Möbius' text. When read in light of this passage, Möbius' pamphlet becomes a clear depiction (and justification) of the metaphorical and spiritual rape to which Elberskirchen refers. Möbius' text is precisely the destructive and demeaning force that, according to Elberskirchen, is rooted in male (hetero) sexual drives and cripples women. What Möbius describes as inborn female feeble-mindedness is a result of the century-long metaphorical and spiritual rape. She stresses, however, that the influences of this violent act manifest themselves not only in the lives of individual women, but also in culture and civilization as a whole.

Elberskirchen points to the following implications of the ideology underlying Möbius' text: it is the position of powerlessness and subjugation that defines women and the position of power and domination that defines men. As soon as a woman attempts to emancipate herself and gain social independence, according to Möbius she ceases to be a woman and becomes "ein Mann mit einem Uterus" (Möbius, *Schwachsinn* 41). By the same token, the rhetoric Möbius uses in his text helps justify male violence against women as natural, or even necessary. He explicitly puts women in a position of helplessness, subjugation, and powerlessness. Conversely, he implies that men are inherently in a position of sexual dominance and power. This spectacle of (male) domination and (female) subordination leads me to characterize his text in terms of pornographic imagination.

5.7 From *Weib* to *Frau*: the New Woman

At the beginning of his pamphlet, Möbius comments on the use of language in the debate about women's emancipation:

> Es ist ganz ungehörig, zur Geschlechtsbezeichnung den Ausdruck "Frau" zu verwenden. Frau ist die ehrende Anrede und bedeutet die Herrin, Domina, Dame, aber nach unserem Sprachgebrauche darf nur die Verheiratete als Frau bezeichnet werden. Wenn man von einer Frauenfrage, Frauenversorgung usw. spricht, so meint man vorwiegend die Angelegenheiten der Weiber, die nicht Frau sind, denn die Frauen brauchen nicht versorgt zu werden usw., sondern die Ledigen und die Witwen; man drückt sich also falsch aus. Dem Manne steht das Weib gegenüber, und der Plural heißt nicht die Frauen, sondern die Weiber. Wenn die Weiber sich ihres Namens schämen sollten, so ist das schlimm genug, aber kein Grund, die Sprache zu vergewaltigen. (*Schwachsinn* 25)

This passage exemplifies the phenomenon of language itself becoming a contested sphere in the struggle for and against the re-definition of gender roles. Generally speaking, physicians opposing women's education used the word *Weib* to refer to all women. Supporters of women's emancipation, however, tended to used the word *Frau* when they intervened in the traditional construction of femininity. They used the word *Weib* to refer specifically to the (pseudo) scientific misogynist construction of femininity.[230] At this time, the word *Weib* began to acquire its negative connotations as it was gradually replaced by the word *Frau*. Titles of influential progressive women's magazines such as *Die Frau, Die Frauenbewegung*, or *Dokumente der Frauen* suggest a conscious effort to enforce the use of the term *Frau*. In this context, the following statement by Dohm is of great significance. Referring to Runge's assertion concerning the conditions under which the annihilation of female nature is inevitable, Dohm cites his warning against the effects of women's emancipation: "[d]ie Vernichtung der Weibernatur, falls das Weib die geschlechtliche Sphäre durchbräche" ("Die Ritter" 47). In the context of the public debate about gender differences, "die Vernichtung der Weibernatur" had a double meaning. For Runge, Möbius, and all like-minded, it was equated with the obliteration of the narrow notion of womanhood and consequently with a destabilization of gender relations. For the supporters of women's emancipation, conversely, it carried with it very positive consequences. By destroying "Weibernatur" as a linguistic and mental construct, women would be able to liberate themselves from the limiting notion of femininity.

Dohm evokes the above nexus of gender concepts and their implications when she sums up the arguments against medical education for women: "[a]uf Grund ihrer physischen Beschaffenheit, auf Grund der Menstruation, Schwangerschaft, Geburt und ihren Folgeerscheinungen kann und darf *die Frau* nicht Medizin studieren!" ("Die Ritter" 34; emphasis added). While *das Weib*, a culturally constructed woman of the nineteenth century, was not able to study medicine due to the limitations imposed on her by this very construct, *die Frau*, a new gender model, could and should pursue an academic education. Because woman was still believed to be limited and defined mainly by her sexuality, she was denied equal education and employment opportunities. With a shift in this understanding of womanhood, women would enjoy the same rights and privileges as men.

Schirmacher distinguishes two different realities reflected by the designations *Weib* and *Frau*. While *Weib* denotes a focus on "Leidenschaft und Sinn" (Schirmacher, "Die Frauenfrage" 655) and refers to a woman primarily as a sexual being, *Frau* denotes a complete human being that is not reduced to her sexuality; she is "Mensch in erster Linie" (Schirmacher, "Die Frauenfrage" 655). Looking back at women's history in Western Europe, Schirmacher concludes that up to the late nineteenth century, women ("Spezies Weib") were "nach einer [...] gleichbleibenden Richtung hin gezüchtet worden" in order to fulfill male fantasies about "das Ewig-Weibliche" which meant primarily "Schönheit, Schwäche, Unterordnung [...]" (Schirmacher, "Die Frauenfrage" 656). She recognizes that the turn

230 Such a use of the terms *Weib* and *Frau* was a strong tendency, but it was not a norm.

of the twentieth century is, indeed, a turning point in the development of social constructions of gender and claims that a new type of female identity is materializing at this time: "[D]ie Frau hört auf, *nur Weib* zu sein, und in der Gattung Weib, die bisher allgemein die einzig anerkannte war, bildet sich eine neue Art: die 'Frau' im eigentlichen Sinne, die 'moderne Frau'" (Schirmacher, "Die Frauenfrage" 655). She further characterizes the New Woman[231] as follows:

> Diese "moderne Frau" ist nicht die Frau der Decadence, der Überreife und Überkultur, nicht die Frau, wie sie Bourget und Maupassant schildern: das Kind flatternder Geselligkeit, des Salons, der Mode, des geschäftigen Müßigganges. – *Sie ist in erster Linie eine geistige Arbeiterin.* In der Literatur ist sie bisher fast noch gar nicht geschildert, wenigstens noch nicht naturwahr und ganz durchgeführt, und im Leben ist sie auch noch nicht anerkannt, sondern sucht sich erst ihren Platz zu erwerben. (Schirmacher "Die Frauenfrage" 655; emphasis added)

Schirmacher hints at fin-de-siècle constructions of femininity, such as the *femme fatale* and the *femme fragile*, that haunt the literary landscape of the time. She also recognizes, however, that these prevalent figures do not reflect the New Woman whose main characteristic is intellectual work. It is quite remarkable that, indeed, literary and artistic representations of female intellectuals are almost non-existent in the canonical literature and male-created culture at the turn of the twentieth century.

Schirmacher also points out that the type *Frau* is not an entirely new phenomenon as it had manifested itself throughout the course of history. She asserts that "die Gattung Weib immer und immer wieder Individuen hervorgebracht [sic], die über das Weib hinaus, die Entwicklung der Frau einschlugen" ("Die Frauenfrage" 657). These, according to her, included women who were financially independent and enjoyed a certain amount of autonomy ("die Königin von Saba," "eine Reihe ägyptischer Prinzessinnen, die Seherin Kassandra, die Brusterin Veleda"), women-warriors ("Judith bis zu Jeanne d'Arc und Charlotte Corday"), artists and writers ("Sappho"), all women who pursue higher education ("die sich durch geistige Arbeit unabhängig machen"), and also the precursors of the nineteenth-century women's movement ("manche von den 'Hexen' des Mittelalters ist nur eine wissensdurstige Frau gewesen und gleich den alten Kräuterfrauen und den Hebammen eine Vorläuferin der modernen Ärztin") (Schirmacher, "Die Frauenfrage" 657-58). What made these women different was their pursuit of roles

231 Thorson discusses representation of the New Woman in fiction written by women in late-nineteenth century; specifically she focuses on Grete Meisel-Hess' novel *Fanny Roth* 211-229. Thorson points out that the female characters representing the New Woman were often juxtaposed with other female characters labeled as "Halben" (211). This juxtaposition is similar to the opposition between *Weib* and *Frau.*

outside of the conventional female one as wife and mother. While the type *Weib* was forced to live a one-dimensional life, the new type *Frau* struggled to gain spiritual, intellectual, or heroic dimensions traditionally unavailable to her; in so doing, she subverted gender boundaries.

Olberg, too, acknowledges the emergence of a new female identity at the turn of the twentieth century. She claims that the traditional virtues such as "der intellectuelle Dämmer, religöse Hingabe, schlichte Frömmigkeit" (Olberg 108) have lost their appeal and actuality. Besides, they have not helped women create a better existence for themselves. She calls these virtues "Gretchentugenden" (Olberg 108) and argues that they had only supported women's subjugation throughout the centuries and had prevented women from acquiring a better social position and autonomy. Instead, they only provided for "die Angst der Unorientiertheit" (Olberg 108). She admits that it is not easy to transform these conditions and mind sets that have existed for centuries, but she believes that it is her generation's mission to change women's inferior status. Olberg claims that the profound technological changes that took place in the nineteenth century had a direct impact on middle-class women because they resulted in women's "Arbeitsentlastung" which, in turn, led to "einer geringeren Verwendung weiblicher Arbeitskraft in der Hauswirtschaft" (Olberg 66). This development created an "Ueberschuss an Kraft" in households, a surplus that could be utilized in intellectual activities (Olberg 67). She claims that prior to the technological advancements of the nineteenth century, such a surplus of female energy did not exist because "bei der starken Inanspruchnahme durch die Fortpflanzungsarbeit und die Hauswirtschaft wenig Kraft übrig blieb" (Olberg 65). In addition, increasing opportunities to access cultural products and education resulted in a new intellectual environment for women:

> Dann hat sich aber auch in der Umgebung, in der sich das Weib normalerweise bewegt, eine Aenderung vollzogen. Schule, Bibliotheken, Vorträge, vor allem aber die Tagespresse haben wie ein weitverzweigtes Gefässystem Anregungen und Wissensfragmente in alle Schichten getragen. Sie haben gleichsam ein neues geistiges Milieu geschaffen, das vielgestaltig und wandelbar ist. Das Weib verlangt danach, sich in diesem Milieu zu orientieren. (Olberg 67)

Olberg's claim regarding the surplus of female energy is not very convincing. The technological advancements of the Industrial Revolution did not have such a profound impact on child-rearing and housework typically performed by a middle-class wife in the late nineteenth century. Her argument concerning new intellectual stimuli and opportunities for women is much more compelling. Olberg also maintains that these new prospects made women aware of the potential available to them outside of the traditional confines of family life. Moreover, according to Olberg, women of the late nineteenth century are inevitably exposed to a number of new stimuli: "Anregungen sind überall vorhanden, [...] man braucht nicht mehr auszuziehen, das Neue zu suchen: es dringt zu uns auf unzähligen Wegen" (85). Olberg connects modernity to an unstoppable multitude of impulses, but she also relates this phenomenon to middle-class women's intellectual emancipation. According to her, the late nineteenth century created not only opportunities for women that did not exist before, but also new demands and, therefore, a change from *Weib* to *Frau* is inevitable.

In light of these statements, the turn of the twentieth century seems to be the Kantian Enlightenment for women. Richarda Huch developed this idea as she discussed the ways in which intellectual work transformed women's lives. According to her, the admission of women to universities marked a new era because female students served as a pioneering force in the development of the concept of the New Woman. Studies at a university gave young women two impulses necessary for this change: unlimited access to knowledge and free interactions with people. Consequently, the female student entered the world as it was known to men. This experience would necessarily transform women and enrich their personalities. Huch characterized the development of the New Woman as follows: "Von zwei Seiten fließt jetzt studierenden Mädchen der neue Lebensquell: der Einblick in die Wissenschaften erschließt ihr die geistige Welt; die Berührung mit Mensch und Leben entwickelt ihre Persönlichkeit und weckt ihren Sinn für die Welt der Dinge" (Huch 743). University education enriches the lives of women and allows them to liberate themselves from the limitations of a traditional female existence. Like Huch, Olberg acknowledged the importance of discovering new cognitive and intellectual dimensions for women:

> Was ihm [dem modernen Weibe] Not thut, ist Erkenntnis [...], die [...] eine weite Lebensauffassung ermöglicht, eine klare Einsicht in das Thun und Treiben der Menschen und seine Gebundenheit an allgemeine Gesetze, jene Einsicht aus der die Milde quillt und das thätige Erbarmen. Ohne ehrliche, geistige Arbeit wird das keinem. Allein auf die natürliche Intelligenz gestellt und das, was ihr fünf gesunde Sinne aus dem beschränkten Kreise der Alltagserfahrung zutragen, kann niemand zu einem Ausblicke kommen. Man muß Stufen hinauf, muß Kenntnisse erwerben. (107)

Hence, pursuing the new cognitive and ontological dimensions is a transformative force and provides opportunities not only for intellectual development, but also for personal growth. It cannot, however, be cultivated in the solitude of the household and without intellectual endeavors. To participate in this pursuit, women demand access to higher education. In other words, the New Woman (*Frau*) leaves behind what Olberg calls "halbbewusste[s] Leben" and embraces "Intellectualismus" (108).

Conclusion

Progressive intellectuals, writers, and activists responded directly to texts opposing academic education for women written by physicians and scientists not only to discredit their arguments, but also to use them as springboards to promote a new understanding of femininity. By critiquing the male-oriented notions of femininity and by focusing on the development of woman's intellectual potential, on her personal fulfillment and satisfaction, on financial independence, and on autonomy in making decisions, the early feminists negotiated new meanings for the female body. While certain male physicians and scientists regarded women as being literally trapped by and in their bodies, the early feminist writers located the woman's self both in the body and outside of it. Hence, the female body became a topic of public discussions and a battleground for cultural and social transformations.

Most of the women responding to the dominant discourse on the female body and sexuality acknowledged their pioneering role and the importance of their work. They recognized their responsibility to speak up in order that change might occur. Dohm explained the motivation underlying female responses to the gender discourse: "Da aber vorläufig die Majorität meiner deutschen Zeitgenossen das Recht der Frau an wissenschaftlichem Beruf leugnet, so dürfen wir kleine Minorität nicht müde werden, für unsere Überzeugung zu kämpfen" (*Emancipation* 8). Binder pointed out that due to the writings supporting the cause of female education, the number of opponents was continuously shrinking and the number of supporters growing (2). Weber also believed that women would be able to study medicine and practice in the medical profession in Germany only if "durch eine lebhaftere Agitation der Frauen selbst die Vorurteile dagegen noch mehr überwunden sein werden" (45). Weber admitted that she wrote her book, *Ärztinnen für Frauenkrankheiten. Eine ethische und sanitäre Notwendigkeit*, with the intent to gain support for female medical education and to give the issue positive publicity. Her book is described as "eine Bitte um Hilfe [...] an alle, die unser Geschlecht hochschätzen" (Weber 46).

In addition to campaigning for support, female authors, through their writings, informed the public in depth about the issue of higher education. They provided accurate statistical data and examples of women's successes in other countries, uncovered women's history, delivered convincing arguments, and, most importantly, called attention to unequal gender relations. Weber, for example, explained that the success of the women's movement depended on a thorough comprehension of female demands and their causes (46). Such an understanding of the issue was possible only through active female participation in the public discussion of women's admission to medical schools and an open exchange of ideas. Likewise, Lange emphasized the importance of the female voice: "Es ist die Frau, die den Mann für die Frauenfrage gewinnen müßte. Diese liegt den Berufswegen der meisten Männer weit ab. Was ihnen davon zu Ohren kommt, ist so zufälliges, unzusammenhängendes Stückwerk, daß sie sich gelangweilt oder auch amüsiert oder empört davon abwenden" (*Frauenbildung* 102).

Women responding to antagonistic pamphlets, speeches, and books were very proficient in arguing that female admission to medical schools was a necessity and that women were capable of intellectual work. What strikes today's reader of the texts supporting women's higher education is the remarkable erudition of their authors, their very skilled argumentation, and their pioneering perspective on gender. Such sophistication enabled these writers to discredit their adversaries, show logical fallacies in their argumentation, prove that they used incorrect or incomplete data, and reveal the hidden grounds of opposition to women's education. They also called attention to the fact that the issue of higher education for women was not a struggle limited to selected individuals. Instead, it related to all women, because it required a re-definition of femininity if a new social order based on gender equality was to be established. Therefore, as Lange put it, "Es werden um dieser Sachlage willen die Frauen sich zu einem Kampf entschließen müssen, der durchaus nicht in ihrer Natur liegt, der aber um ihres eigenen Geschlechts willen zur Gewissenssache wird" (*Frauenbildung* 34). Considering the traditional, very limited, and mind-numbing education of middle-class girls at that time, it is remarkable that these female authors were able to liberate themselves intellectually, at least to a certain degree, from the long-established gender norms and to gain such a deep knowledge in so many fields. As I have argued throughout this book, many of the texts written in support of higher education for women in the late nineteenth century foreshadow various aspects of contemporary feminist theory and issues addressed by gender and women's studies in the late twentieth century.

Works Cited

Albert, Eduard. *Die Frauen und das Studium der Medizin.* Wien: k.u.k. Hof- und Universitäts-Buchhändler, 1895.

Asmus, Martha. "Ein Retter vom Geist. Antwort auf die Schrift des Herrn P.J. Möbius: 'Der physiologische Schwachsinn des Weibes.'" *Die Gesellschaft* 17.2 (1901): 232-240.

Avicenna (Fritz Wittels). "Weibliche Ärzte." *Die Fackel* 3 Mai 1907: 10-24.

Bandhauer-Schöffmann, Irene. "Frauenbewegung und Studentinnen. Zum Engagement der österreichischen Frauenvereine für das Frauenstudium." *"Durch Erkenntnis zu Freiheit und Glück..." Frauen an der Universität Wien (ab 1897).* Ed. Waltraud Heindl and Marina Tichy. Wien: Universitätsverlag, 1990. 49-78.

Bartky, Sandra Lee. "Foucault, Femininity, and the Modernization of Patriarchal Power." *The Politics of Women's Bodies. Exuality, Appearance, and Behavior.* Ed. Rose Weitz. New York: Oxford UP, 2003. 25-45.

Bäumer, Gertrud. "Die Mädchenbildung im 19. Jahrhundert." *Handbuch der Frauenbewegung.* Ed. Helene Lange and Gertrud Bäumer. 5 vols. Berlin: W. Moser Buchhandlung, 1901-1906. 3: 72-128.

Beruna, Anna. *Darf die Frau denken?* Minden: n.p., 1893.

Binder, S[idonie]. *Weibliche Ärzte, Eine Studie.* Stuttgart: Göschen'sche Verlagshandlung, 1892.

Bischoff, Theodor. *Das Studium und die Ausübung der Medizin durch Frauen.* München: Literarisch-Artistische Anstalt, 1872.

"Bluestocking." *Encyclopaedia Britannica.* 2001 Deluxe Edition CD-ROM.

Bornemann, Regina. "Erste weibliche Ärzte. Die Beispiele der 'Fräulein Doctores' Emilie Lehmus (1841-1932) und Franziska Tiburtius (1843-1927). Biographisches und Autobiographisches." *Weibliche Ärzte. Die Durchsetzung des Berufsbildes in Deutschland.* Ed. Eva Brinkschulte. Berlin: Edition Hentrich und bei dem Institut für Geschichte der Medizin der Freien Universität Berlin, 1993. 24-32.

Borostyani, Marie. *Das Recht der Frau. Vermächtnis einer Unglücklichen and ihre Mitschwestern. Gedanken und Vorschläge aus dem Nachlaß einer Verstorbenen.* Zürich: Verlags-Magazin. (J. Schabelitz), 1885.

Brinkschulte, Eva, ed. *Weibliche Ärzte. Die Durchsetzung des Berufsbildes in Deutschland.* Berlin: Edition Hentrich und bei dem Institut für Geschichte der Medizin der Freien Universität Berlin, 1993.

Brinkschulte, Eva. "Dr. med. Maria Daelen. Ein Titelbild und die Lebensgeschichte einer engagierten Ärztin." *Weibliche Ärzte. Die Durchsetzung des Berufsbildes in Deutschland.* Ed. Eva Brinkschulte. Berlin: Edition Hentrich und bei dem Institut für Geschichte der Medizin der Freien Universität Berlin, 1993. 5-10.

Brook, Barbara. *Feminist Perspectives on the Body.* London: Longman, 1999.

Brühl, Marie. *Die Natur der Frau und Herr Professor Runge.* Leipzig: Hermann Seemann Nachfolger, 1903.

Brunner, Margit. "Sexualle Gewalt gegen die Studentinnen um die Jahrhundertwende." *Signale, Veröffentlichungen zur historischen und interdisziplinären Frauenforschung* 1 (1994): 75-97.

Brupbacher, Fritz. *Geburtshelfer Runge und die Frauen-Emanzipation.* Zürich: Speidel, 1899.

Büchner, Ludwig. "Das Gehirn der Frau." *Die Frau* 1 (1893/94): 308-314.

Bülow, Frieda Freiin von. "Das Weib in seiner Geschlechtsindividualiät." *Die Zukunft* 18 (1897): 596-601.

---. "Schwachsinn des Weibes." *Die Zukunft* 37 (1901): 13-19.

Burchardt, Anja. "Die Durchsetzung des medizinischen Frauenstudiums in Deutschland." *Weibliche Ärzte. Die Durchsetzung des Berufsbildes in Deutschland.* Ed. Eva Brinkschulte. Berlin: Edition Hentrich und bei dem Institut für Geschichte der Medizin der Freien Universität Berlin, 1993. 10-21.

Busch, Regine. "Neues für und wider die Frauen." *Der Türmer. Monatsschrift für Gemüt und Geist.* 4.1 (1901-1902): 71-75.

Caputi, Mary. *Voluptuous Yearnings. A Feminist Theory of the Obscene.* Lanham: Rowman & Littlefield Publishers, 1994.

Cauer, Minna. "Die Wissenschaft und die Frauenbewegung." *Die Frauenbewegung* 1 Feb. 1896: 26-27.

Connel, R. W. *Masculinities.* Berkeley: U of California P, 1995.

Digby, Anne. "Women's Biological Straitjacket." *Sexuality and Subordination.* Ed. Susan Mendus and Jane Rendell. London: Routledge, 1989. 192-220.

Dijkstra, Bram. *Idols of Perversity. Fantasies of Feminine Evil in Fin-de-Siècle Culture.* New York: Oxford UP, 1986.

---. *Evil Sisters. The Threat of Female Sexuality in Twentieth-Century Culture.* New York: Henry Holt and Company, 1996.

Diprose, Rosalyn. *The Bodies of Women. Ethics, Embodiment and Sexual Difference.* London: Routledge, 1994.

Dohm, Hedwig. *Die wissenschaftliche Emancipation der Frau.* Berlin: Wedekind & Schwieger, 1874.

---. "Die Ritter der *mater dolorosa.*" *Die Frauenbewegung* 15 Feb. 1897: 33-36.

---. "Die Ritter der *mater dolorosa.*" *Die Frauenbewegung* 1 Mar. 1897: 45-48.

---. "Randglossen zur Schrift 'Über den physiologischen Schwachsinn des Weibes' von P. J. Möbius." *Die Frauenbewegung* 1 Feb. 1901: 18-20.

---. "Randglossen zur Schrift 'Über den physiologischen Schwachsinn des Weibes' von P. J. Möbius. Fortsetzung." *Die Frauenbewegung* 15 Feb. 1901: 26-28.

---. "Randglossen zur Schrift 'Über den physiologischen Schwachsinn des Weibes' von P. J. Möbius. Schluß." *Die Frauenbewegung* 1 Mar. 1901: 35-36.

Dworkin, Andrea. *Pornography: Men Possessing Women.* New York: Perigee Books, 1981.

Elberskirchen, Johanna. *Feminismus und Wissenschaft.* Leipzig: Magazin Verlag Jacques Hegner, 1903.

Ellis, Havelock. "Das Gehirn der Frauen." *Die Zukunft* 9 (1894): 128-136.

Fausto-Sterling, Anne. *Myths of Gender. Biological Theories about Women and Men*. New York: Basic Books, 1985.

---. *Sexing the Body. Gender Politics and the Construction of Sexuality*. New York: Basic Books, 2000.

Freudenberg, Ika. "Oda Olberg contra Dr. Moebius." *Die Frau* 9 (1901/1902): 620-626.

Frevert, Ute. "Bürgerliche Meisterdenker und das Geschlechterverhältnis. Konzepte, Erfahrungen, Visionen and der Wende vom 18. zum 19. Jahrhundert." *Bürgerinnen und Bürger. Gerschlechterverhältnisse im 19. Jahrhundert*. Ed. Ute Frevert. Göttingen: Vandenhoeck u. Ruprecht, 1988. 17-48.

Friedman, Steve. "Down with Love." *Elle* May 2004: 166-168.

Glaser, Edith. "'Sind Frauen studierfähig?' Vorurteile gegen das Frauenstudium." *Geschichte der Mädchen- und Frauenbildung*. Ed. Elke Kleinau and Claudia Opitz. 2 vols. Frankfurt/ New York: Campus Verlag, 1996. 2: 299-309.

---. "Die erste Studentinnengeneration – ohne Berufsperspektiven?" *Geschichte der Mädchen- und Frauenbildung*. Ed. Elke Kleinau and Claudia Opitz. 2 vols. Frankfurt/ New York: Campus Verlag, 1996. 2: 310-324.

Griffin, Susan. *Pornography and Silence*. New York: Harper & Row, 1981.

Gumplowicz, Ladislaus. "Polemisches zur Frauenfrage." *Sozialistische Monatshefte* 8.11 (1904): 901-913.

Hainisch, Marianne. *Seherinnen, Hexen und die Wahnvorstellungen über das Weib im 19. Jahrhundert*. Wien: Verlag der "Deutschen Worte," 1896.

---. "Die Geschichte der Frauenbewegung in Österreich." *Handbuch der Frauenbewegung*. Ed. Helene Lange and Gertrud Bäumer. 5 vols. Berlin: W. Moser Buchhandlung, 1901-1906. 1: 167-188.

Heindl, Waltraud. "Zur Entwicklung des Frauenstudiums in Österreich." *"Durch Erkenntnis zu Freiheit und Glück..." Frauen an der Universität Wien (ab 1897).* Ed. Waltraud Heindl and Marina Tichy. Wien: Universitätsverlag, 1990. 17-26.

---. "Aspekte des Wandels?" *"Durch Erkenntnis zu Freiheit und Glück..." Frauen an der Universität Wien (ab 1897).* Ed. Waltraud Heindl and Marina Tichy. Wien: Universitätsverlag, 1990. 151-152.

---. "Exkurs: Die russischen Studentinnen an der Wiener Universität. Ein Beispiel ausländischer Hörerinnen." *"Durch Erkenntnis zu Freiheit und Glück..." Frauen an der Universität Wien (ab 1897).* Ed. Waltraud Heindl and Marina Tichy. Wien: Universitätsverlag, 1990. 129-136.

---. and Marina Tichy. "Einleitung: Fragen, Methoden und Quellen." *"Durch Erkenntnis zu Freiheit und Glück..." Frauen an der Universität Wien (ab 1897).* Ed. Waltraud Heindl and Marina Tichy. Wien: Universitätsverlag, 1990. 9-15.

Heinsohn, Kirsten. "Der lange Weg zum Abitur: Gymnasialklassen als Selbsthilfeprojekte der Frauenbewegung." *Geschichte der Mädchen- und Frauenbildung.* Ed. Elke Kleinau and Claudia Opitz. 2 vols. Frankfurt/ New York: Campus Verlag, 1996. 2: 149-160.

"Hetaera." *Encyclopaedia Britannica.* 2001 Deluxe Edition CD-ROM.

Hoesch, Kristin. "Die Kliniken weiblicher Ärzte." *Weibliche Ärzte. Die Durchsetzung des Berufsbildes in Deutschland.* Ed. Eva Brinkschulte. Berlin: Edition Hentrich und bei dem Institut für Geschichte der Medizin der Freien Universität Berlin, 1993. 44-55.

Huch, Richarda. "Über den Einfluss von Studium und Beruf auf die Persönlichkeit der Frau." *Gesammelte Werke. Fünfter Band. Gedichte, Dramen, Reden, Aufsätze und andere Schriften.* Köln, Berlin: Kiepenheuer&Witsch, 1971. 743-755.

Ichenhaeuser, Eliza. *Die Ausnahmestellung Deutschlands in Sachen des Frauenstudiums.* Berlin: Verlag von Hermann Walther, 1897.

---. "Die Frauenstudienfrage in Deutschland." *Die Kultur* 2 (1903): 1052-1058.

Jentsch, Ernst. "Zur Erinnerung an Dr. P.J. Möbius" and "Einführung." P.J. Möbius. *Beiträge zur Lehre von den Geschlechts-Unterschieden.* Halle: Verlag von Carl Marhold, 1907. 5-31.

Kappeler, Susanne. *The Pornography of Representation.* Cambridge: Polity P, 1986.

Kirchhoff, Arthur, ed. *Die Akademische Frau. Gutachten hervorragender Universitätsprofessoren, Frauenlehrer und Schriftsteller über die Befähigung der Frau zum Wissenschaftlichen Studium und Berufe.* Berlin: Hugo Steinitz Verlag, 1897.

Kohler Riessman, Catherine. "Women and Medicalization. A New Perspective." *The Politics of Women's Bodies. Exuality, Appearance, and Behavior.* Ed. Rose Weitz. New York and Oxford: Oxford UP, 2003. 46-63.

Krause, Christianne. "'Hetärismus' und 'Freie Liebe' gegen 'Bürgerliche Verbesserung': Franziska zu Reventlow in den 'Zürcher Diskussionen.'" *Lulu, Lilith, Mona Lisa...Frauenbilder der Jahrhundertwende.* Ed. Irmgard Roebling. Pfaffenweiler: Centaurus-Verlagsgesellschaft, 1989. 77-98.

Kronfeld, M. *Die Frauen und die Medizin. Professor Albert zur Antwort. Zugleich eine Darstellung der ganzen Frage.* Wien: Verlag von Carl Lonegen, 1895.

Lange, Helene. *Frauenbildung.* Berlin: L. Dehmigke's Verlag, 1889.

---. *Higher Education of Women in Europe.* Trans. L.R. Klemm. New York: D. Appleton and Company, 1890.

---. "Professor Albert und das medizinische Studium der Frauen." *Die Frau* 3 (1895/96): 145-148.

---. "Die akademische Frau." *Die Frau* 4 (1896/97): 193-199.

---. "Frauenlogik." *Die Frau* 5 (1897/1898): 516-522.

---. and Gertrud Bäumer, ed. *Handbuch der Frauenbewegung.* 5 vols. Berlin: W. Moser Buchhandlung, 1901-1906.

Laqueur, Thomas. *Making Sex. Body and Gender from the Greeks to Freud.* Cambridge: Harvard UP, 1990.

MacKinnon, Catharine A. *Feminism Unmodified. Discourses on Life and Law.* Cambridge: Harvard UP, 1987.

"Maenad." *Encyclopaedia Britannica.* 2001 Deluxe Edition CD-ROM.

Martin, Emily. *The Woman in the Body. A Cultural Analysis of Reproduction.* Boston: Beacon P, 1987.

Mayreder, Rosa. "Zur Physiologie des weiblichen Geschlechtes" *Dokumente der Frauen* 1 (1899): 66-69.

---. "Die schöne Weiblichkeit." *Dokumente der Frauen* 1 (1899): 119-125.

Mazón, Patricia M. *Gender and the Modern Research University. The Admission of Women to German Higher Education, 1865-1914.* Stanford: Stanford UP, 2003.

McDowell, Linda, and Joanne P. Sharp, ed. *Space, Gender, Knowledge. Feminist Readings.* London: Arnold, 1977.

Meyer, Heinrich. "Professor Runge und die Frauen." *Die Frau* 6 (1899): 710-716.

Michels, Robert. "Das Weib und der Intellectualismus." *Dokumente der Frauen* 7 (1902): 106-114.

Möbius, Paul Julius. *Über den physiologischen Schwachsinn des Weibes.* München: Matthes & Seitz Verlag, 2000.

---. *Beiträge zur Lehre von den Geschlechts-Unterschieden. Nebst einer Einführung von Dr. Ernst Jentsch und einer biographischen Skizze.* Halle: Verlag von Carl Marhold, 1907.

Morawski, Jill G. "Femininity." *Women's Studies Encyclopedia.* Ed. Helen Tierney. 2002 Greenwood Publishing Group, Inc. 17 Mar. 2005 <http://gw2.scbbs.com/wse/wse.jsp?l=F&id=id227>.

Morgenstern, Lina. *Ein offenes Wort über das medizinische Studium der Frauen an Herrn Prof. Dr. W. Waldeyer.* Berlin: Verlag der deutschen Hausfrauen-Zeitung, 1888.

Niranjana, Seemanthini. *Gender and Space. Femininity, Sexualization and the Female Body.* New Dehli: Sage Publications, 2001.

"Notizen." *Dokumente der Frauen* 1 (1899): 42.

Olberg, Oda. *Das Weib und der Intellectualismus.* Berlin: Akademischer Verlag für sociale Wissenschaften, 1902.

Parons, Clare Olivia. "Reputation and Public Appearance: The De-Eroticization of the Urban Street." *Voices in the Street. Explorations in Gender, Media, and Public Space.* Ed. Susan J. Drucker and Gary Gumpert. Cresskill, New Jersey: Hampton P, 1997. 59-70.

Paul, H. *Die Überschätzung der Jungfernschaft. Ein Beitrag zur modernen Frauenfrage*. Dresden: Verlag H. L. Diegmann, [1905?].

Pollock, Griselda. *Vision and Difference. Feminism, Femininity and the Histories of Art*. London: Routledge, 1988.

"Pornography." *Oxford English Dictionary.* Oxford UP 2005. 20 Mar. 2005 <http://dictionary.oed.com/cgi/entry/50184353?single=1&query_type=word&queryword=pornography&first=1&max_to_show=10>.

"Pornography." *The Barnhart Dictionary of Etymology.* Ed. Robert K. Barnhart and Sol Steinmetz. United States of America: H. W. Wilson Company, 1988.

Raschke, Marie. "Wissen verdummt." *Die Frauenbewegung* 1 Apr. 1895: 51.

---. "Die weibliche Ehre." *Die Frauenbewegung* 15 Dec. 1897: 250-251.

Rohner, Hanny. *Die ersten 30 Jahre des medizinischen Frauenstudiums an der Universität Zürich 1867-1897.* Zürich: Juris Druck + Verlag Zürich, 1972.

Runge, Max. *Das Weib in seiner geschlechtlichen Eigenart.* Berlin: Verlag von Julius Springer, 1904.

---. *Männliche und weibliche Frauenheilkunde.* Göttingen: Vandenhoeck & Ruprecht, 1899.

Schiebinger, Londa. *Has Feminism Changed Science?* Cambridge, Massachusetts: Harvard UP, 1999.

Schiller, Francis. *A Möbius Strip. Fin-de-Siècle Neuropsychiatry and Paul Möbius.* Berkeley: U of California P, 1982.

Schirmacher, Käthe. "Die Frauenfrage." *Die Gesellschaft. Monatschrift für Literatur, Kunst und Sozialppolitik* 1894: 651-661.

---. "Die akademische Frau." *Die Frauenbewegung* 1 Jan. 1897: 2-4.

---. "Die akademische Frau." *Die Frauenbewegung* 15 Jan. 1897: 15-17.

---. "Die akademische Frau." *Die Frauenbewegung* 1 Feb. 1897: 27-28.

Schmaußer, Beatrix. *Blaustrumpf und Kurtisane. Bilder der Frau im 19. Jahrhundert*. Stuttgart: Kreuz Verlag, 1991.

Schmersahl, Katrin. *Medizin und Geschlecht. Zur Konstruktion der Kategorie Geschlecht im medizinischen Diskurs des 19. Jahrhunderts*. Opladen: Leske + Budrich, 1998.

Schmidt, Hedwig. "Randbemerkungen zu der Broschüre von Prof. Möbius." *Hamburgische Schulzeitung: eine Wochenschrift für pädagogische Theorie, Kunst, und Erfahrung.* 14 (1906): 408-409.

Sontag, Susan. "The Pornographic Imagination." *Styles of Radical Will.* New York: Farrar, Straus and Giroux, 1969. 35-73.

Spain, Daphne. *Gendered Spaces*. Chapel Hill: U of North Carolina P, 1992.

Steinem, Gloria. "If Men Could Menstruate." *Outrageous Acts and Everyday Rebellions.* New York: Henry Holt and Company, 1995. 366-369.

Stolle, Rosa. *Sklavenketten der Frauen.* Leipzig: Verlag von Max Spohr, 1893.

Sveistrup, Hans, and Agnes v. Zahn-Harnack, ed. *Die Frauenfrage in Deutschland, Strömungen und Gegenströmungen 1790-1930, Sachlich geordnete uns erläuterte Quellenkunde*. N.p.: August Hopfer Burg, 1934.

Theweleit, Klaus. *Male Fantasies*. 2 vols. Minneapolis: U of Minnesota P, 1996.

Thorson, Helga Mae. "Re-Negotiating Borders: Responses of German and Austrian Middle-Class Women Writers to Medical Discourses on Sex, Gender, and Sexuality at the Turn of the Century." Diss. U of Minnesota, 1996.

Tichy, Marina. "Die geschlechtliche Un-Ordnung. Facetten des Widerstands gegen das Frauenstudium von 1870 bis zur Jahrhundertwende." *"Durch Erkenntnis zu Freiheit und Glück..." Frauen an der Universität Wien (ab 1897)*. Ed. Waltraud Heindl and Marina Tichy. Wien: Universitätsverlag, 1990. 27-48.

---. "Soziale Herkunft, Elternhaus und Vorbildung der Studentinnen." *"Durch Erkenntnis zu Freiheit und Glück..." Frauen an der Universität Wien (ab 1897)*. Ed. Waltraud Heindl and Marina Tichy. Wien: Universitätsverlag, 1990. 93-107.

Troll-Borostyáni, Irma von. "Etwas über Weiblichkeit." *Die Frau* 1 (1893/94): 811-813.

---. "Heilfrauen – statt Ärztinnen." *Die Frauenbewegung* 15 Nov. 1895: 175-177.

Tuma, Renate. "Studienwahl – Fächerwahl – Studienabschlüsse." *"Durch Erkenntnis zu Freiheit und Glück..." Frauen an der Universität Wien (ab 1897)*. Ed. Waltraud Heindl and Marina Tichy. Wien: Universitätsverlag, 1990. 79-92.

Ussher, Jane M. *Fantasies of Femininity: Reframing the Boundaries of Sex.* London: Penguin, 1997.

"Vestal Virgin." *Encyclopaedia Britannica.* 2001 Deluxe Edition CD-ROM.

Waldeyer, Wilhelm. "Das Studium der Medizin und die Frauen." *Tageblatt der Versammlung Deutscher Naturforscher und Aerzte* Sept. 1888: 31-44.

Walker, Lynne. "Home and Away. The Feminist Remapping of Public and Private Space in Victorian London." *New Frontiers of Space, Bodies and Gender.* Ed. Rosa Ainley. London: Routledge, 1998. 65-75.

Weber, Mathilde. *Ärztinnen für Frauenkrankheiten. Eine ethische und sanitäre Notwendigkeit.* Berlin: Dehmigke's Verlag, 1893.

Weiershausen, Romana. *Wissenschaft und Weiblichkeit. Die Studentin in der Literatur der Jahrhundertwende.* Göttingen: Wallstein Verlag, 2004.

Wytek, Rudolf. "Anhang: Statistiken und Graphiken." *"Durch Erkenntnis zu Freiheit und Glück..." Frauen an der Universität Wien (ab 1897).* Ed. Waltraud Heindl and Marina Tichy. Wien: Universitätsverlag, 1990. 153-187.

Ziegeler, Beate. *Weibliche Ärzte und Krankenkassen. Anfänge ärztlicher Berufstätigkeit von Frauen in Berlin 1893-1935*. Weinheim: Deutscher Studien Verlag, 1993.

---. "'Zum Heile der Moral und der Gesundheit ihres Geschlechtes...' Argumente für Frauenmedizinstudium und Ärztinnen-Praxis um 1900." *Weibliche Ärzte. Die Durchsetzung des Berufsbildes in Deutschland*. Ed. Eva Brinkschulte. Berlin: Edition Hentrich und bei dem Institut für Geschichte der Medizin der Freien Universität Berlin, 1993. 33-43.

Berliner Beiträge zur Literatur- und Kulturgeschichte

Herausgegeben von Irmela von der Lühe und Gail K. Hart

Band 1 Magdalena Tarnawska: ...*und Medea war eine Ärztin*. Constructions of Femininity in Public Debates about Medical Education for Women in Germany and Austria between 1870 and 1910. 2007.

www.peterlang.de